before
& after

Living & Eating Well
After Weight Loss Surgery

SUSAN MARIA LEACH

WILLIAM MORROW
An Imprint of HarperCollins*Publishers*

This book is dedicated to my husband, Ty, who loves me for my heart no matter what size I am; and to my mother, Beatrice, who I wish were here to share my happiness. I can now look in the mirror and find her smile in my face.

HarperCollins books may be purchased for educational, business, or sales promotional use. For information please write: Special Markets Department, HarperCollins Publishers Inc., 10 East 53rd Street, New York, NY 10022.

FIRST EDITION

Designed by Jennifer Ann Daddio

Printed on acid-free paper

Library of Congress Cataloging-in-Publication Data

Leach, Susan Maria.
    Before & After : living & eating well after weight loss surgery / Susan Maria Leach.—1st ed.
        p. cm.
    Includes bibliographical references and index.
    ISBN 0-06-056722-8
        1. Leach, Susan Maria—Health.   2. Gastric bypass—Popular works.   3. Overweight women—United States—Biography.   I. Title.

RD540.5.L43   2003
362.1'96398'0092—dc22
[B]

                                                                                                2003059384

         06   07   08   WBC / RRD   10   9   8   7   6   5   4

contents

acknowledgments   v

foreword by dr. carlos carrasquilla   vii

a note from a nutritionist   xi

preface   xiii

introduction   1

the countdown to june 11 begins!   13
    preoperative journal

june 11, 2001 . . . my post-op life begins!   17
    postoperative journal

questions and answers
about weight loss surgery   61

protein, carbohydrates, and sugar
after weight loss surgery   85

protein shakes   93

soups, purees, and other soft foods   102

fish and seafood   125

chicken and turkey   157

desserts   191

cooking for the holidays   224

sources   245

index   253

acknowledgments

Thank you to Dr. Carlos Carrasquilla for caring enough to perfect this amazing surgery.

Special thanks to:

Ronni, for being my best friend and knowing when to give me that gentle nudge to take action, whether in a mall buying shoes or when wrestling with the decision to have weight loss surgery.

John, who I will admit, is as good a cook as I am (except for Key lime pie). I would not have taken a picture of a speedometer while driving at a ridiculously high rate of speed on the autobahn for anyone but you.

Daddy and Diane, for taste testing all of my sugar-free desserts on Sundays. I love you both.

Nicholas . . . hmmmm, Sue and Nick's Spicy Pretzel Sticks. Awesome, it's in my next book.

Stephanie, who gave me competition to goal weight, and is my muse for anything sugar-free and chocolate.

Jo, for having the guts to make a change. I am so happy for your new life and that you allow me to be a part of it.

Harriet, for recognizing how many people this project will help and for allowing me to keep my own voice. I am lucky to be working with you.

foreword

DR. CARLOS CARRASQUILLA

Obesity is a worldwide epidemic, and is rampant in the United States. It is newly-recognized as a major disease. The problem of obesity is not merely the individual's physical appearance, but also the health risks and ultimately the increased incidence of death. To know that in the United States alone, there are more than 300,000 preventable deaths yearly, about thirty-four each hour, is very serious and frightening.

There is a considerable list of diseases called *co-morbidities* associated with obesity, which aggravate an already serious situation. The co-morbid complications could be psychological, social, economic, and, of greater concern, medical. The list includes illnesses such as diabetes, hypertension, coronary artery disease, respiratory problems, reflux, and an extended sub-list of illnesses with different degrees of seriousness. The gravity of the health status varies with the increase of weight in the individual.

To the patients with a status of "morbid obesity"—100 pounds or more above their ideal weight—the treatment of choice becomes surgery, since non-surgical methods are projected to have an almost total failure rate. Several procedures have been used for weight control. The most common procedure today is the gastric bypass, considered the "gold standard of bariatric surgery."

Historically, we have used different types of surgery to obtain and maintain weight loss. We have created malabsorption, physical restriction of the intake of food, and a combination of these two procedures, with variations developed by individual surgeons. Currently we are investigating electrical impulses to the muscles of the stomach to produce the feeling of satiety.

The results after gastric bypass surgery have been extraordinary, not only with the appearance of the patient, but also with improvement or correction of the health risks. In our center, together with my partners, Drs. Wayne English and Paul Esposito, I have been very happy with the results during the last few years. The average excess weight loss at twelve months post-op has been to 82 percent in over 1400 patients on whom we have operated. Among the patients with diabetes, 93 percent of them have stopped taking medication and enjoy normal blood sugar levels. Of the hypertensive, 84 percent of patients have returned to normal blood pressure levels, allowing them to discontinue their medications. Other problems such as sleep apnea have also been corrected or improved.

Patients such as Susan, who are interested in improving their quality of life both physically and emotionally, come to us for information to help them achieve their goals. Those who meet the criteria for bariatric surgery and make the decision to proceed on this journey are given a road map to guide them through. Should they choose to continue to move forward, they will have a surgical consultation and psychological and medical clearance. Once this has been accomplished they proceed with surgery and are on the road to a healthier, happier, and slimmer life. As they approach each crossroad, the decision as to which road to take ultimately becomes theirs.

In the practice of bariatric surgery, with the establishment of dedicated and specialized centers, the great majority of the patients have an ongoing patient-physician relationship. The patients' relationships to each other are also fascinating; they bond together in a fraternity, exchanging information and assistance. It gives us great pleasure and becomes a source of pride to see the changes in these patients, not only in their obvious physical development but also in their health status and new, self-confident personalities.

With Susan, we have seen her radiance and beauty reflected in the eyes of her admiring husband. Her energetic personality exudes assurance, confidence, and the enthusiasm of someone who wants to share her positive experience with others in her situation. Susan relates the story of her life and at the same time, organizes this book to help other patients in that fraternity to facilitate their further success and happiness. Since Susan has personally made that journey, it was her desire to assist her fellow travelers on their way. Realizing that adaptation to certain dietary requirements may be more difficult for some than others, Susan has written this excellent and much-needed book.

In her diary, Susan tells readers how she handled her range of emotions from her decision to undergo surgery to the panic she felt when taking her first drink of water, to later, when she could enjoy only small portions of decadent meals while traveling. Through her encouragement and her recipes, Susan shows how others can discover the pleasures of cooking and eating while maintaining their dietary limitations.

Susan's book shows people who are used to big, rich, and indulgent meals how to adapt their cooking to include healthier choices without losing flavor or feeling deprived. In *Before & After* Susan teaches the reader how to make the necessary dietary changes from Day 1 post-op. Starting with protein shakes, and moving on to "Soups, Purees, and Other Soft Foods," she progresses to more elaborate meals while at the same time maintaining the crucial nutritional requirements. Other patients can discover and enjoy the pleasure of cooking while maintaining the limitations of the "rules of the game."

At one of our regular support group meetings, Susan delighted the members with samples of her low-carbohydrate desserts. As the desserts disappeared before my eyes, I couldn't help noticing the reactions of the group members, who expressed pleasure and surprise in knowing they can enjoy good food without hindering their progress or compromising their health.

If you are considering obesity surgery, my advice is to find an established, dedicated, specialized center with experienced surgeons who provide adequate follow-up with dietary and psychological support. Insist that the surgeon and the team educate you on all aspects of this disease and treatment. Then, they should prepare themselves for the lifetime adjustments necessary for successful completion of their goal. By arming yourself with Susan's book, you will find the journey a lot more pleasurable.

—Carlos Carrasquilla, M.D., F.A.C.S., director, Florida
Center for Surgical Weight Control, P.A.

A Note from a Nutritionist

In the fast-growing area of gastric bypass surgery, new information on the subject is vital. As a dietitian in a bariatric surgeon's office, I have worked with over 400 gastric bypass patients this year alone. There is a clear need for more appetizing advice on how to prepare foods post-operatively that will appeal to people. Having this surgery should not and does not mean that once-loved foods can no longer be enjoyed. This book is full of recipes to create meals and treats that are tastier than the foods many people may have had even prior to surgery.

When I reviewed the book and its recipes, I was seeing it from a nutritional perspective. I was very impressed (and a little surprised) with how well the recipes align with the guidelines developed by the American Society of Bariatric Surgery. These recipes are prepared without the addition of sugar, which is restricted in the bypass patient due to the adverse reaction it may cause. Susan Leach is conscientious of the carbohydrate content of the foods that are prepared. This is important because carbohydrates are restricted in the post–gastric bypass patient, making it easier to get in much-needed protein. Many of her recipes are also high in protein, which is a staple of the post–gastric bypass diet. While this book was written with the gastric bypass patient in mind, it can be used by anyone looking for delicious recipes that promote a healthy weight and lifestyle.

—Jennifer Pereira, RD, LD/N

preface

When I had my successful gastric bypass surgery on June 11, 2001, I landed with both feet firmly planted in my new world with no turning back. I decided from the start that I wasn't going to prepare special meals for myself; I was going to come up with dinners for my entire family. This book is the map of my travels and discoveries in cooking.

Everyone in these times wants to eat healthier foods in smaller portions, so without realizing it, my entire circle of family and friends had signed on for this ride. Since I am a creative cook, it has been easy for me to come up with ways to prepare foods that are not only full of protein and low in fat and carbohydrates, but also absolutely delicious. I have changed my relationship with food, but I didn't have to leave my favorite ingredients and piquant flavors behind!

There are many foods that are very easy to eat after this surgery, but some will always be difficult. Add in the fear of not chewing well enough, worries about "dumping," panicking about stretching our new pouch, and it is no wonder that finding something to eat can be a major problem during the first twelve-month post-op period. Certain food textures work well, and lower fat sauces to moisten the foods are a must.

In addition to more than 100 recipes in this book, there are ideas to help the post-op cook stay on the path and adapt his or her own recipes. I've also included tips for eating out and cooking during the holidays. There is an introduction to protein, carbohydrates, and sugar for those who are post-gastric bypass surgery, as well as a list of sources for special foods and ingredients.

It is now almost three years since my surgery and I have happily melted down to a size 8. I weigh 135 pounds and I am ecstatic to have lost more than one half my original body weight. I find myself at the beginning of a new life. More important is the fact that I feel fantastic and I am healthier than I have been in years! Life as a bariatric gourmet is pretty fabulous.

introduction

About a week before the life-altering bariatric surgery that would reduce my stomach to the size of a small egg, I found an envelope containing a folded, yellowed letter, neatly printed in pencil, in a box of family pictures. I had written it to my wonderful Great-Aunt Rose when I was 6 years old. Although it was precious to her, she had given it to my mother to save for me.

May 30, 1968

Dear Aunt Rose,

How are you and your family? We are all fine at home. This is my first letter to anyone. Mother helped me with the hard words. I get all A's on my report card. I am in the first grade. Grandpa said I could come to Florida with them next time to visit you. We will leave Johnny at home he's always crying for Mother . . . Dad is nice and skinny he lost 47 lbs of fat. Mom is skinny too. Johnny is skinny and I am getting tall. See you soon.

Love, Susan

I have always joked that I wasn't too heavy, I just wasn't tall enough; apparently I had already figured this out when I was in first grade. The words in the letter make me laugh, but clearly I was dealing with weight issues even as a six-year-old. I had analyzed my entire family and felt that I needed to justify myself; they weren't just thin, they were *skinny*. Did someone tell me not to worry about my weight because I would be getting taller sometime soon? Instead of pretending with my Barbie or playing on my swings, I was waiting to get tall.

I suffered from the usual assortment of childhood humiliations: innocently asking what the letters "OW" meant next to my second-grade weight of 91 pounds and having the school nurse loudly announce to a room full of my classmates that it stood for overweight; not being able to zip my powder blue one-piece gymsuit in Catholic grade school. Gym class was a source of terror throughout my school life in general, particularly the uneven parallel bars during a junior high gymnastics rotation. I stood in the back of the group afraid to even twitch; the sympathetic gym teacher mercifully lost track of me for a couple of weeks. There was a minor bright spot: two other fat girls in my class ranked even lower than I did since *they* couldn't throw or hit a ball, so at least I avoided the horror of being chosen last for teams. I overheard my best friend's older sister laughingly tell the cute new boy in town (and object of my summer crush) that I was a "baby blimp." At first I had no inkling that she was talking about me, but as the realization crept over me I felt the warm flush of shame as I stood in their kitchen. In fourth-grade English class, what were the odds that one of the spelling words of the day, *obese*, would correspond to my unfortunate choice of seat, where I had to stand up, correctly spell *and* use the word in a sentence? In grade school and junior high my father affectionately called me "Chubbette" and "Chubby." I still prefer to tell myself that it was simply his little term of endearment, and that he would have never used the pet name if he thought he was hurting me, but in retrospect it does seem insensitive. These incidents are just a few that stand out in my mind; every fat person has his or her own repertoire of similar stories. I wouldn't want to go back in time to change them—who knows what I would be like today without these character builders?

I tried everything to lose weight. My mother took me to Weight Watchers meetings when I was 10. I have taken turns with Cambridge, Slimfast, Optifast, total food deprivation, Atkins, hormone injections, bizarre cabbage and banana régimes, hospital-supervised programs, and a nasty bout with bulimia in college while trying to keep off weight I had starved myself to lose for a spring break trip. I would typically lose 20 pounds, then lose control and gain back 25 pounds. For most of my adult life, I have carried between 200 and 235 pounds on my medium 5-foot, 7-inch frame. Several years ago when I easily lost 32 pounds in two short months courtesy of the prescription weight-loss drugs fenfluramine and phentermine, commonly known as Fen-Phen, I thought these medications were finally going to be the thing that worked. Many of my friends were also taking this combination of pills that made it a breeze to push away the half-eaten plate of food, and we were a very happy group of losers. When the media storm about the side effects of fenfluramine and phentermine appeared, I decided that I was finished torturing myself with unhealthy diets. I convinced myself that being healthy and heavy were not mutually exclusive, and I could be both. I rationalized that I was fighting nature and that I should be happy the way I was meant to be. I always wore beautiful clothes and was meticulous about my hair and makeup. People knew I was competent and confident in business. I was happy, funny, I had an incredible husband, a great marriage, and now that I decided that I was not going to live within the restraints of dieting, I was finally free.

Over the next three years, I slowly but steadily ballooned to 278 pounds. I was now bursting out of 26/28, the largest size sold at Lane Bryant. The 3X sizes at Bloomingdale's were tight, and I became completely disgusted with what I had done to myself by eating whatever I wanted. My neck and chest were so large that I was having trouble breathing when I would lie in bed. A custom, handmade sterling silver necklace that was a prize vacation purchase in Taxco, Mexico, now choked me. I couldn't even pretend I weighed less by creatively standing on one foot on the sweet spot on my scale. The cute, chubby little girl was now a morbidly obese 39-year-old woman; the "pretty face" was now distorted by fat into a face that I couldn't recognize in a mirror. For a few months I was actually thinking that the changes in the appearance of my face were a function of my approaching fortieth birthday rather than my approaching 300 pounds. When I started noticing that I didn't fit into booths at too many restaurants for it to be a coincidence, and I couldn't get my hair cut by John, my favorite stylist at In Sync because their zippered smocks didn't fit my increasing girth, I made more and more excuses to stay home. I spoke with my best friend, Ronni, on the phone almost daily, but didn't make the fifteen-minute trip to her home for over eight months. At my largest weight, I only left home to shop for groceries. I had few clothes that fit me, and I would stay in my silk bathrobe until late afternoons on most days. I was too humiliated by the smock situation to get my hair cut so I let it grow down to the middle of my back and rarely, if ever, made up my face anymore. I had so many "headaches" on days we were to attend parties and events that my husband suggested that I see a neurologist. As I got larger my world became very, very small.

In February 2001, I saw the image that changed my life: the newly-svelte Carnie Wilson, Beach Boy Brian Wilson's daughter and member of the pop group Wilson Phillips, on the cover of *People* magazine. Carnie was standing with both of her legs in one leg of her "fat" jeans, wearing a petite, bright red peasant blouse, beaming with pure joy. I read that article over and over and was amazed by the weight loss operation that I had previously only heard of in passing. The operation is called the Roux-en-Y Gastric Bypass procedure, commonly known as RNY. Even though the procedure was quite involved and the article stressed that it was major surgery, it didn't seem radical to me, since Carnie's procedure was done laparoscopically through five tiny incisions. Carnie had learned about the procedure while appearing on Roseanne's show, when the comedian shared that she had lost almost 100 pounds after having gastric bypass surgery the previous year. Carnie researched the details, made her decision, and with the support of her family and friends, went ahead with the surgery, even broadcasting parts of the procedure on an Internet site. After losing almost half of her body weight she was proudly showing off her physique in the pages of *People*.

I could relate to Carnie Wilson's story. As each of Wilson Phillips's hits was released with a video, Carnie was heavier and less prominently featured. She had a breathtakingly beautiful face, yet they tried to keep her body hidden and minimize her appearance in each song while Wendy Wilson, her extremely thin sister, and Chynna Phillips writhed around in lingerie. I was so embarrassed for her, and felt as if I were the only person who understood what she was going through. Seeing Carnie on that magazine cover and reading her story brought me to tears. I was so happy for her and for the hope that this surgery gave me. It was my defining moment: I realized how miserable I was at 278 pounds and decided that I had to do something about it.

I jumped on the Internet and started gathering every bit of information I could find about the Roux-en-Y Gastric Bypass operation. The stomach is reduced to a thumb-sized pouch, from which the remainder of the stomach is divided with multiple rows of staples and permanently separated. The small intestine is cut about eighteen inches below the stomach, then pulled up and attached to the new small stomach pouch. The larger, lower portion of the stomach is bypassed, but still provides digestive gastric juices for the small intestine. The small size of the pouch effectively stops the patient from eating too much at any given meal, while the bypassed intestine somewhat diminishes the ability to absorb the food that *is* eaten. A few ounces of food constitute a meal, and the sheer volume restriction on food intake is the first mechanism of weight loss. One or two small bites beyond satisfaction will create a stuffed feeling. A small bite beyond that will cause discomfort and nausea, and yet another small bite will cause pain and subsequent vomiting. The gastric reduction also works by creating satiety, the feeling of being comfortably full and satisfied. Filling the pouch with a small meal feels the same as if the whole stomach had been filled with a very large Thanksgiving feast.

The pressure against the stomach walls triggers nerve signals that travel to the appetite center of the brain to give the feeling of satisfaction. Even though the portion size is small, there is no hunger and no feeling of having been deprived. People who have had this surgical procedure no longer live to eat, they eat to live. In other words, the gastric bypass surgery not only alters the anatomy for capacity, but also modifies how the brain's appetite center functions.

The best way to look at this procedure is to understand and visualize that the surgeon is creating a pouch, and this pouch is a tool to be used by the patient to control his or her weight. The surgery is not magic, and it can be a disaster if a patient expects the procedure to remove the weight automatically without changing his or her relationship with food. There is no jumping off the wagon for a holiday meal or special occasion. Bariatric surgery is not an easy way out for weight loss, as there are many potential trade-offs and changes in lifestyle. You have to accept the fact that you can *never again* gorge yourself on a multi-course meal of appetizer, salad, bread, Porterhouse steak with a loaded baked potato, cappuccino, and a crème brûlée. You have to deal emotionally with the fact that you can *never* eat all of anything, no matter how good it tastes. Physically, you can no longer eat more than a couple of ounces of tender filet mignon, two or three bites of a vegetable, and a small taste of the dessert. Early on, I just kept repeating my new mantra "Nothing tastes as good as thin feels!" Within a few months of surgery, it came true.

To be considered a candidate for the procedure, you must be clinically morbidly obese. Morbid obesity marks the point where the disease begins to interfere with your basic physiological functions such as breathing, walking, and sleeping. It is defined as the condition of weighing two or more times your ideal weight; however, a more accurate indicator is having a Body Mass Index (BMI) of 40 (kg/m^2) or greater. BMI is a calculation that relates an individual's weight to their height. The ideal BMI is between 19 and 25. If you have a BMI of between 25 and 30, you are considered to be overweight. At a BMI of

30 or over, you are considered obese. A BMI of 40 or more indicates severe or "morbid" obesity. Morbid obesity increases the complications of pregnancy, surgery, and injuries, and the incidence of breast and uterine cancers in women, prostate cancer in men, and colon cancer in both. "Super morbid obesity" is defined as 200 percent over ideal body weight, about 320 pounds for women and 360 pounds for men; it exponentially increases the incidence of disease, injuries, and early death. Gastric bypass surgery is only presented as an option for those whose weight is high enough that the medical risk of their obesity outweighs the risks of the procedure.

The RNY procedure is considered to be the most effective operation, offering the best combination of maximum weight loss with minimum nutritional risk for the morbidly obese. The top bariatric surgeons agree that it is the best available operation at this time in terms of *safety*, with less than a 0.5 percent mortality rate with surgeons who are trained in this procedure, even taking into consideration that these patients are high risk operative candidates; *effectiveness*, with patients averaging an 80 percent loss of excess weight at one year; and fewer undesirable *side effects* for the patient, meaning minimal vomiting, the ability to eat a wide selection of healthy normal foods, and no chronic intestinal difficulties. More than 98 percent of all weight-related health problems or co-morbidities are relieved by one year after the operation—usually within weeks.

The RNY gastric bypass procedure can be done using an open technique gaining access to the abdomen through a single large midline incision, or as a laparoscopic procedure. With laparoscopic surgery, the surgeons prepare the patient by inserting a series of tubes called *trocars* into tiny incisions. These tubes serve as channels through which the surgeon inserts a pencil-thin fiber-optic camera, which projects an image onto a television screen; a device to inflate the body cavity with gas to essentially float the organs apart; and long instruments with tips that cut, grip, and staple. It is an amazing and complex skill for a surgeon to master. The advantages to the patient are enormous: less pain, a shorter hospitalization, and a quicker return to normal life. Most of the post-op pain comes not from the organs operated on, but from the layers of skin, fat, and muscle tissue that were cut to gain access to them. Few surgeons are skilled in this highly specialized method of surgery, so finding a laparoscopic surgeon who performs the RNY gastric bypass operation can be a challenge in some parts of the country. Now that this procedure has grown in popularity, it is more important than ever to investigate the facts of this surgery, become an expert on how your body will be affected by this operation, the risks and benefits as they pertain to you, and the background of the surgeon to whom you are entrusting your life. When flying on a commercial airliner you want a skilled and practiced pilot in the cockpit; when having this surgery, whether laparoscopic or open, you want a skilled and practiced surgeon with an established track record, who performs this procedure frequently.

After taking in mountains of information, I summoned my best friend, Ronni, and tentatively explained the surgery to her with the help of the Spotlight Health website (www.SpotlightHealth.com). We spent the entire day at my computer looking at before-and-after pictures, reading Carnie's narrative of her procedure, reading other peoples' accounts of their surgery, and discussing the actual procedure. I brought in a big basket of Doritos to snack on while we calculated our BMIs on the website. Size 4 Ronni came in at a whopping BMI of 19 kg/m^2, while mine was almost 41 kg/m^2. Since I didn't have any medical conditions such as diabetes or hypertension to heighten my need for the procedure, my BMI had to be over 40 for me to even be considered for the surgery. Ronni pushed the Doritos toward me and said, "Here, eat these!" We laughed at the irony of my needing to maintain my preoperative weight. It appeared that I was actually the perfect candidate for the RNY gastric bypass procedure. Gaining support from my wonderful husband, Ty, would be simple once I had the details ironed out.

I would not be alone in taking this permanent surgical step to solve my lifelong battle with weight. In 2001, more than 47,000 people had gastric bypass surgery. In 2002, more than 63,000 opted for the surgery, the number more than doubling since 1999. This year the number is expected to surge to over 120,000. More people are coming out and letting us know of their weight loss surgery successes. The latest additions to the growing list are *The View*'s Star Jones, *American idol* judge Randy Jackson, and author Anne Rice, who is best known for her best-selling novel *Interview with a Vampire*. They are on the heels of *Today* show weatherman Al Roker, who openly discussed his procedure after the nation witnessed his steady plunge from 320 to less than 190 pounds since March of 2002. Singer Ann Wilson, of Heart, underwent her bariatric procedure in January 2002 and now chronicles her progress on Spotlight Health right beside Carnie Wilson. The front man for the band Blues Traveler, John Popper, went from over 420 pounds to a slim 185 after his RNY surgery in 2000. The NBC-TV series *Ed* worked 500-pound actor Michael Genadry's gastric bypass procedure into their storyline for the 2003 season. Do you think that the Osbornes would have ever had a shot at MTV and mainstream stardom with a 250-pound, morbidly obese TV mom? Probably not! The now-diminutive Sharon Osborne had her gastric procedure in 1999 and is enjoying incredible celebrity as the glue that holds this unconventional family together. Increasing numbers of public figures are announcing their successes with RNY surgery, thus creating an even bigger demand all over the country.

I needed to locate a bariatric surgeon to perform my surgery. I was very fortunate to find qualified laparoscopic bariatric surgeons where I live in South Florida. I scheduled my consultation with Dr. Carlos Carrasquilla for March 15, 2001. After completely disclosing all aspects of the procedure and giving me a thorough physical, Dr. Carrasquilla said that I was an excellent candidate for the laparoscopic procedure. I felt comfortable placing my future in his expert hands; his levels of confidence, skill, and experience were overwhelming, and gave me the strength to make my final decision. With my approval to go ahead, his staff scheduled my surgery for June 11, 2001.

Now that I had a date for surgery, I had plenty of time to second-guess myself. My only hesitation was in regard to cooking and lifestyle. I absolutely love to cook and have been a "foodie" forever. I have always subscribed to *Gourmet* and *Bon Appétit* magazines. I have my TV tuned into The Food Network at least six hours a day. I have aged balsamic vinegar in my kitchen along with chipotle peppers, wasabi powder, pure ancho chiles, tahini, fish sauce, twenty-eight bottles of hot sauce, a quart bottle of Sriracha, a chunk of imported Parmigiano-Reggiano, and containers of oil-cured olives. My husband and I love to travel to Mexico, where I comb local markets in search of dried chiles, freshly made tortillas, and unusual fruit. Everywhere we go we sample local cuisine—ceviche, jerk pork, Pilsner beer, fiery salsas, hand-pressed olive oils, Black Forest ham, and cracked conch. Ty and I also collect agave tequila. On a trip to Germany, my goal was to track down a source of local homemade cherry liqueur, Kirschwasser. I love to make dinner and entertain at our home. I have baked magical candy-covered gingerbread houses for more than 25 years; it wouldn't be Christmas without them.

Food has always been a part of my life and even though I was committed to changing my body and eating habits for better health, I didn't want to totally give up my lifestyle. Food is part of who I am. I didn't want to be thin and miserable; I didn't want to have to exist on special food while we traveled the world. I didn't want to be the freak eating the soup. So now that I had a surgical answer, I wanted to see if I could exist as an RNY gourmet.

I learned from other people who had RNY surgery that we can eat normal food once we are past the first 7 to 8 months post-op, just in much smaller amounts. Everyone said their tastes and cravings changed somewhat after surgery, and they now eat healthier foods. I discovered that those enjoying hot, spicy, and bold flavors, like me, still enjoyed them post-op. I talked to people at their goal weight who loved to cook before their surgery, and still loved to cook after their surgery. What I learned from those who had undergone surgery was that food had to be moist to be easy to eat and digest. In addition, sugar was no longer an option with the new configuration of our intestines, but with Splenda, Nutrasweet, and other sugar-free innovations, I could enjoy creative desserts and satisfy that occasional urge for a few bites of pie.

There was no reason why I wouldn't be able to travel, cook for my friends and family, and still enjoy cookbooks, Emeril Lagasse on television, and my subscription to *Gourmet* after my surgery. It was just going to take planning, experimentation, and dedication to a new way of eating.

the countdown to june 11 begins!

May 26, 2001

I feel so weepy and emotional. I went to breakfast this morning with my husband, my father, and his wife, and I sat there staring at my plateful of scrambled eggs, fried potatoes, sausage, and bagel slathered with cream cheese; it made me feel so terrible about myself, I wanted to cry. I couldn't eat it. Lately, I analyze what is on my plate at every meal and think, "I will never eat this again." It is a very difficult feeling to deal with. Then five minutes later, I get angry with myself and think, "You have eaten enough in your life, get over it!" I regroup my thoughts and it is more like "I will never eat this much for one meal or on one plate again!"

June 5, 2001

My best friend, Ronni, and I checked out the surgical floor at Florida Medical Center. The fifth-floor bariatric suites appeared comfortable and clean. It made me feel so much better about the surgery looming before me. Everyone I have come in contact with at this hospital has been exceptional. When they perform a diagnostic test, the technicians are very professional and know what they are doing, and there is no confusion. You can feel so exposed and vulnerable in this setting, but the staff has given me even more confidence in my choice. The nurses took the time to talk to me and showed us around the floor, even taking us into one of the specially-equipped bariatric rooms. I was surprised to see that this hospital has large leather recliners, and the beds have a steel frame canopy with a hanging bar you can use to help move yourself. I will be in a private room. Ronni will stay with me the first couple of nights since my husband can be pretty useless in medical situations, and I mean that in a loving way. I adore my husband, but after I had throat surgery two years ago, it took him entirely too long to figure out that my frantic hand gestures meant I desperately needed some water.

I have been comparing notes with people on the weight loss surgery message boards and some of their hospitals and surgeons don't have scales capable of weighing them, or compression stockings to fit their large legs, or even hospital gowns for larger patients. I wonder why someone would choose a surgeon or hospital that didn't make special accommodations for the comfort and safety of larger patients. More importantly, I wonder why a bariatric surgeon specializing in this procedure would not make sure that his or her hospital provided these items for their patients.

I only have a few days left to eat "big food" so tonight we are going out for pizza. Tomorrow, Ruth's Chris Steak House is on the calendar so that I can enjoy a final giant steak. I am 39 years old and I figure that I have eaten enough. I will be able to eat again, albeit in very small portions, but I will enjoy a few more days of shameless gluttony. I am scared, but on most days I can't wait to get rolling.

June 8, 2001

I am looking forward to being on the "losing" side of this surgery. Tonight, my husband went solo to a party we were invited to. The invitation touts that there will be a band with dancing, cocktails, and incredible food. I just didn't want to go. I am the biggest that I have ever been in my life, so of course my first thoughts were of my closet full of clothes too tight to wear. My newest size 26/28 Lane Bryant jeans are so tight that if that button on the waistband popped, the ricocheting metal could injure an innocent bystander. I can barely breathe while sitting down in them. My black knit twin set, the only acceptable item in my closet for a casual party, will make my makeup run in ten minutes flat in the humid June night air. Everyone will be running around in little tops and mini skirts and I would be the red-faced fat girl in the hot sweater and jeans. The clincher that cemented my decision to stay home was that it is a yacht christening party and I just know I would have been in an uncomfortable situation getting on and off the boat. I have already had a couple of embarrassing situations on friends' boats! Even when you can get on the boat, you have to worry about the tide changing. On one occasion a fairly easy two-foot jump down to the boat later became an impossible four-foot leap back up to the dock. I immediately recognized the problem at hand and watched in terror while everyone else seemed to fly effortlessly up to the dock aided by the helping hands of the uniformed boat valets. I tried to think of a reason to stay on the boat, but there was no way out. When my husband and a friend's husband realized that I was going to have difficulty getting up to the dock, they began to formulate a plan to help me. Then more of our friends became aware that there was a problem and got back on the boat to help. I found myself the sudden focus of attention while our well-meaning friends pulled and pushed me upward. As my feet landed on the dock, I tried to act nonchalant about whose hands had been on my butt, giving me that final boost. I suffered not only from embarrassment, but also large bruises on my arms and legs from the incident. This was supposed to be a fun end to a day of boating, but I remember it for the humiliation instead of the event we were celebrating.

Tonight, our dear friends giving the party will wonder where I am. I tried to beat it into my husband's head that information was to be given out strictly on a need-to-know basis. He is allowed to tell only those who asked that I am having my gallbladder removed on Monday. I am so sad to send him off by himself, but I have comfort in knowing that this is the last time.

before

June 10, 2001

I am spending this last night before my surgery reading the on-line journals of people who have had weight loss surgery. There are so many women who are the same age, height, and weight as I am, that I am able to get a pretty reasonable picture of what to expect. After reading at least 100 stories and clicking on hundreds of before-and-after pictures, I am at peace with the whole thing. I have eaten my last meal of Sunday morning blueberry pancakes drenched with butter and drowning in real Vermont maple syrup. Now I can only have clear liquids until midnight and then nothing by mouth. I feel as if I am in a plane with my parachute carefully packed.

june 11, 2001 . . . my post-op life begins!

June 22, 2001

My surgery was much tougher than I expected. Other patients from the same day were in and out in three days; my procedure took longer than usual and involved a great deal of tugging and pulling to get my parts where they needed to be. If I hadn't had such an experienced surgeon, my laparoscopic RNY would have turned into an open RNY. I am lucky that Dr. Carrasquilla has had other tough cases. This proves my theory that you don't need a great surgeon for a routine procedure, you need one in case your procedure produces the unexpected. In addition, my intestines didn't quite "wake up" from the surgery for a few days, creating lots of trapped gas. So, after the first days of feeling as if I had been hit by a large truck, I quickly recovered and spent the rest of my hospital time feeling fine (considering that I just had my guts rearranged), but waiting to blow out the gas! The nurses not only took great care of my physical needs but also knew how to handle my vulnerability. I had a longer hospital stay than most and they knew how disappointed I was about it. The nurses couldn't have been more wonderful; I just didn't expect to stay with them for 9 days for a laparoscopic procedure.

This is my third night at home. I am still very uncomfortable with these staples—I am afraid they will catch on something. My stomach is swollen and somewhat bruised. I look like a manatee with my huge, bloated belly. The five cuts scattered across my belly are a strange sight. I am scheduled to have the staples removed tomorrow. The water and broth that I am constantly sipping is going down easily. I have not had any trouble at all with nausea or vomiting. I have an over-all feeling of fullness and although I am not hungry, I made myself eat several small bites of food each day since I am sure that my body needs protein after all it has been through. A protein shake is easy for me to eat and takes a good half an hour to consume. The creamy, cold, banana protein shake I make every morning makes me feel very full. I sit at my computer sipping my shake instead of coffee while I read my e-mail. I can feel it trickling down into my stomach as the coldness spreads downward. How odd. Cold and thick seems to work better than a thin liquid shake.

My family is coming over for a barbeque this weekend. I plan on making some pinto bean puree, a large salad, and grilled turkey burg-ers; a feast for all and I can eat a small portion of beans, since I am restricted to eating soft foods. I am beginning to understand the lifestyle changes I will need to make.

June 25, 2001

I am healing very well and I feel great. My only complaint is that I have one spot that pulls and burns when I get out of bed from a flat posi-tion. I am still eating pureed foods like egg custard and sugar-free pud-ding, and I have not had any problems at all. I have a second protein shake in the afternoon since I need the protein to heal. If I can just eat small portions of normal foods, this will be easy. I had my staples removed on Friday and it didn't even pinch. It seems that the holes from the staples are worse than the incisions. I have seven little cuts, actually five little cuts and two drain holes . . . twenty-one staples in all but nothing that some Neosporin won't heal. I was afraid to get on the scale at the doctor's office because of all the bloat I still have in my belly, but the surgical assistant cajoled me and I have lost 16 pounds. Ta da! I was shocked.

July 7, 2001

So here I am at 25 days post-op, and just getting back to feeling good again! The food situation is revealing itself. At first, I didn't understand why I didn't really get a full feeling with very soft foods. I was worrying that my pouch may have been fashioned in too large a size. Now that I am eating more solid items, feeling full sneaks up on me! I measure out my little portions of food for my plate and sometimes I can get only halfway through those small amounts. I am through before I am ready to be! Soups, custards, and tuna salad taste the best and go down easily. I didn't understand other people talking about foods being moist when I was pre-op, but the other day when I made turkey burgers on the grill, after three small bites I felt as though I had eaten three pounds of burger and it was all backed up in my chest. The feeling was very unpleasant, so I pushed food around on my plate so my family didn't question me. I don't want my surgery to put me in the spotlight, which is why I had everyone over for dinner in the first place. Good thing I made pinto bean puree with a little light sour cream and cheddar on top, it was delicious. My favorite egg salad doesn't taste good anymore. Oddly enough I am finding that I don't care what or if I am eating. I never thought that this would happen to Food TV's number one viewer.

My husband is talking about taking a trip to the Mirage in Las Vegas. I had to laugh because my first thought was that my breakfast days of prime rib, jumbo shrimp, and bagels smeared with cream cheese and piled high with smoked salmon are over! I can't believe that my first thoughts are of the food I will be missing. It goes to show you that it takes a while for your head to catch up with your body after this procedure. Then I had wonderful thoughts of being able to buy a gorgeous blouse or pair of pants in one of those expensive "thin people's" boutiques, or being able to buy the David Yurman bracelet that I want with my winnings and not having to settle for the only one that fits my large wrist. On this next trip things will be different! I told Ty that I will play blackjack in the seat next to him because now I won't keep bugging him that it is time for supper!

July 12, 2001

I am one month post-op! I never thought that I would feel this good so quickly. I walk on the treadmill six days a week and my weight loss is keeping me going. I went to put on a pair of jeans yesterday and they fell off my hips! I couldn't believe it. I had so much swelling and bloat in my lower belly that I couldn't even button the jeans two weeks ago. When I stepped on the scale at the surgeon's office, the nurse put the big weight on 200. I cringed and told her she needed to move it to 250, but then when she slid the small weight over, it balanced at 47. I couldn't believe that I only weigh 247! That is 31 pounds in one month. No wonder my jeans were so loose.

My husband got me going this morning when I put on my baggy jeans. He told me to go to my closet and put all my clothes that are the same size as the baggy jeans in a bag and take them to the church thrift store, since I will never be big enough to wear them again for the rest of my life. How is that for a happy reality moment? I have cleaned out my drawers and my closet and found all kinds of great outfits that will fit again soon! I am thrilled. I am officially happy to have had this surgery. Until now, I vacillated between regret and cautious optimism.

I have been eating fish almost every night without any trouble. Grilled salmon, baked tilapia, or sautéed shrimp, with low- or no-fat sauces for the fish and a very small portion of the vegetables I made for the family. My favorite is mango salsa. I mix finely diced mango with lime juice, cilantro, red onion, and Tabasco, a tablespoon of olive oil, and salt and pepper. It can moisten a piece of fish or even roasted turkey breast, but at this point the fish is much easier for me to digest. I tried a bit of grilled chicken and it didn't seem to go down as well, giving me indigestion and an uncomfortable overstuffed feeling after a bite or two. I will stick to fish and shrimp.

I find that a protein shake is great for breakfast and gives me a much-needed 30 grams of protein. I can see that with as little as I can eat for a meal, I will always have to be conscientious about taking in enough protein. Zero Carb Isopure Creamy Vanilla is the best—with a small piece of banana, skim milk and some ice, it is tasty and smooth to sip.

As far as food—still no nausea or problems. When I woke up from surgery I *never* thought I would ever feel this good again! The scars on my stomach are fine pink dashes and will be gone by the end of the summer. I am slowly melting.

July 23, 2001

I invited my dad and his wife, Diane, for the first spaghetti and meatball Sunday dinner since my operation. It's tough for Italians to go without sauce for six weeks! I made little meatballs so I could have two of them, and I ate two pieces of ziti. I put lots of sauce on top so it was soupy.

The problem came later on when we broke out the Pepperidge Farm cake that my Dad so thoughtfully brought for my husband's birthday. I cut the cake into huge pieces so everyone else would eat it all. I never realized how tough it is to *not* lick your fingers when you cut a layer cake. But I resisted the urge. Actually the prospect of getting sick with "dumping syndrome" in front of everyone in my living room kept my frosting-filled fingers out of my mouth! I had an Eskimo Pie sugar-free fudge pop and although it was chocolaty, it certainly was not Pepperidge Farm cake. Oh well, I am sure it didn't taste as good as thin will feel.

July 30, 2001

Well this is day 49 post-op and my *only* complaint is that I still can't sleep on my stomach. The pain between my belly button and the left incision has finally gone away. I stopped walking for a few days, stopped bending over, stopped twisting my hips, and stopped doing everything that made the pain stab. The doctor checked me out and said it wasn't a hernia, just the nerve endings shooting off until the muscle mends. Some people are just sensitive and have more pain. The lower left incisions are commonly the cause of some distress since this is the site through which most of the surgery is done, and therefore has more muscle tearing and stretching. A few days ago, I woke up and the pain was gone. I have resumed walking again.

Got on the scale and in forty-nine post-op days I have lost 43 pounds. Yesterday, when I ate too fast, I threw up. It is actually better described as regurgitation. It was the same chewed-up mouthful of food I had earlier eaten, but since I do not have stomach acid it was not vile. I had better pay attention and eat slowly. I recall my surgeon explaining that our stomach configuration is like the drain in a sink; if you turn on the water slowly, the water smoothly flows down the drain but if you turn on the water full force, the drain backs up.

I feel fantastic. I have so much energy. I am excited about finding clothes in my closet that fit me again and even more excited about taking my old big clothes to the church thrift store. My goal is to be down 50 pounds in 60 days and I believe that I will make it.

August 8, 2001

I made it through my first post-op sushi experience. My very first *restaurant* experience, actually. We were out having cocktails with friends (I had my bottle of water) and the idea came up to grab some sushi. I was a little nervous but figured I could wing it.

I ordered four thin pieces of tuna sashimi, just the fish slices without rice, and a Florida hand roll: sliced scallops baked with scallions, fish roe, and spicy Japanese mayonnaise rolled into a cone of seaweed. I picked the scallops out of the cone; the sauce made them easy to eat.

I gave Ty two pieces of my tuna, since I was getting full. All in all, a great restaurant experience! Dr. Carrasquilla was right; I have become a cheap date. Our usual $80 sushi tab was just $35 tonight.

August 13, 2001

I don't have an official reading on my doctor's scale until August 21, but unofficially I have lost 53 pounds in nine weeks! I am so excited and I can't believe how fast I am dropping in size. I had better wear some of my smaller clothes quickly or I will miss the opportunity. Even though it seems I am not losing as much weight as in the very beginning I am losing more inches than before. I have lost four sizes.

I am still preparing dinners for my friends and family, who still love my cooking and haven't noticed that everything is lower in fat and carbs. I am still a great cook!

September 16, 2001

I ate some crabsticks for lunch this afternoon and have felt sick ever since. About an hour after I ate them I started feeling terrible. Ty sells real estate and we were showing a million-dollar home to customers when I had to drop back from the group to throw up in the master bathroom. When I lifted the seat on the commode, I realized that the water wasn't hooked up yet. I ran outside and spit up into the bushes. I was so embarrassed. I spent about 40 minutes avoiding my husband and the clients as they toured the home, so they wouldn't see me retching in the shrubbery. I only ate 3 pieces of the stuff and threw up a much greater volume than I consumed. I finally made it home and collapsed on my bed. I tried drinking some water, but that flew out too. I haven't eaten anything that could have blocked my opening. This was not a good day. Note: Susan will not be eating crappy surimi imitation crab ever again!

September 30, 2001

I am so happy about this surgery; it is the best thing I could have done for myself. I am addicted to my scale and weigh myself every morning. I am poised at breaking the 200 mark, but cannot imagine being less than 200 pounds.

I am adding a wider range of soft foods, in small portions. Best of all, eating in restaurants isn't the problem I thought it would be. I went to a birthday party at a restaurant last night and I didn't order my own food, since the portions were so large. I just asked Ronni if I could share hers. Her fish entrée arrived and there were four huge planks of blackened grouper. She would never have been able to eat all of it, and even together we didn't finish the plate. Another friend had an Asian chicken salad and I had some of her greens. It is amazing how everyone is so interested in my surgery, encouraging me to eat off their plates instead of ordering my own. Everyone is paying attention to my new eating habits, watching how little I eat, observing how small I cut my pieces and how long I chew my food. Nothing tastes as good as being thinner feels. I can finally say that with confidence. My clothes are hanging on me. I just bought two shirts in size 18 that are on the verge of being too big for me! I should have ordered a 16 for sure.

October 11, 2001

I just walked in from a wonderful evening out and had to sit down and write about the unabashed happiness I am experiencing. For those of you struggling with your decision to have the surgery, and those of you who have just had their surgery and are struggling with the first few weeks: it all gets so much better! My four-month post-op anniversary is tomorrow and I have lost 79 pounds as of this morning.

Friends who have a membership in the Tower Club, an exclusive private dinner club in downtown Fort Lauderdale, invited us to dinner. The view of the ocean, Intracoastal Waterway, and city lights was breathtaking, the room beautiful, and the staff superlative. The food was excellent. I ate an incredible dinner and stayed within my guidelines.

Cocktails were served in the lounge, hors d'oeuvres accompanied. I had an imported mineral water served in a champagne glass so it would appear that I was having a cocktail. We were then seated in the main dining room with a 360-degree bird's-eye view of the city and ocean. A small square of pâté on rye toast was served as a palate teaser while we looked at our menus. I only nibbled a corner of the pâté, and didn't touch the hot roll placed on my bread plate. I shared a pear and blue cheese salad with raspberries and baby greens with Jayne. I ate slowly and chewed well but consumed less than half of the half portion I was served. Then a palate cleanser of fresh raspberry sorbet was served in a beautiful etched glass dish; much as I would have liked to taste it, I passed, since I was not sure of the sugar content. I knew that sugar could make me sick with the new configuration of my stomach and intestines, and didn't want to test my limits. My entrée soon followed: a whole Dover sole, boned tableside and placed on a platter with a swirl of potato puree, baby green beans, and baby yellow squash. The fish was so fresh and the light lemon, butter, and caper sauce was delicious. I ate most of one half of the fish fillet since protein comes first, skipped the potato carbs, and ate a couple of green beans. The dessert cart was presented. My heart sank as the first plate was set down with a large hunk of a chocolate raspberry cheesecake torte with raspberry coulis, then a slice of mango cake with fruit puree and cream decorating the large platter, and the signature crème brûlée. I sighed and told my friends to order the first one so I could watch them enjoy it. The waiter picked up on my sad tone and asked me why none of the selections pleased me. I stumbled for a second and then mumbled as a cover that I was a diabetic. Without missing a beat he smiled and told me the pastry chef is famous for his sugar-free chocolate chip cheesecake, or would be happy to make me a dish of mixed berries with a sugar-free Romanoff sauce. He said they would serve a sliver, a slice, or a slab. I asked for a sliver of the sugar-free cheesecake and a cappuccino. I tasted my sugar-free cheesecake and was in heaven. It was delicious, but even though it was sugar-free I ate only three small bites since I was full. I sampled one of Ty's blackberries with a dab of the Romanoff sauce. I sipped my cappuccino and enjoyed the rest of the evening smiling broadly, knowing that I had just enjoyed a fabulous dinner that would not prevent me from losing my 80th pound on my four-month post-op anniversary tomorrow! I love what this surgery has done for me and I love my life, my friends, my husband, the way I feel, my new slimmer body in my newly fitting narrow black pants and favorite chartreuse and black lace blouse. Life is excellent and it will get even better.

October 20, 2001

I am getting ready for a 1950s party that we have been invited to attend this evening. It isn't too often that I wear short socks and a skirt that twirls in the air when I spin. I have a custom-made, thick pink felt skirt, appliquéd with a black fuzzy poodle with a rhinestone collar and braided leash, a black twin sweater set, a sheer pink scarf to fasten my ponytail, rolled down bobby socks, black and white Bass saddle shoes and my husband's 1958 class ring on a gold chain for the finishing touch. I splurged and ordered the stiff full crinolines to wear under my skirt. When I put the crinolines on, my skirt is so big I can't get though the door. How am I going to go to the bathroom in this outfit without dunking my skirt in the toilet? I wouldn't have considered going to this party if I hadn't lost this weight. I would have been much too self-conscious to squeeze my 300-pound body into a big pink skirt.

Other than Ty drinking too much tequila and acting like frat boy in front of all our friends, the party was great. I found it was very difficult to find something to eat. The '50s theme featured carhop food. There was a hot dog cart, a large grill with genuine White Castle burgers sizzling away, french fries bubbling in submerged baskets, a cotton candy machine, a popcorn machine, all set up in the enormous courtyard

driveway. Then dinner was served in the "malt shop:" meatloaf, maca-
roni and cheese, green beans, and corn. There was a soda fountain set
up with sundaes and milkshakes, hmmmmm . . . still nothing for me
to eat. I tried to eat a White Castle burger but it was too greasy. The
music was great, and I easily had the most authentic outfit at the party.
No one else had crinolines—they really made my outfit. What fun it is
to dance and twirl around and spin and jitterbug. What a fun party.
Losing this weight is fantastic. I felt so free to dance and have fun. I
could tell that several of our friends noticed that there was something
different about me and made a point of mentioning that I looked great,
but no one attributed it to losing weight. I am not discouraged by this
as these aren't people who see me often enough to notice 80 pounds.

November 3, 2001

Last night we celebrated Ronni's birthday. The plan was for a few
friends to meet at her home and drive to a special restaurant for dinner.
When I arrived at her home I discovered that the plan had changed,
and her cool and stylish mom, Joyce, had hired a stretch limousine to
take all of us to The Blue Door at the Delano in South Beach, Miami.
Dealing with this food challenge will be a real test for me. I am excited
at the idea of eating in this well-known restaurant, but I fear that I will
struggle with the restrictive component of my surgery. Will the happiness I derive from sitting at the table in a smaller size be enough to
compensate for not being able to finish my heaping plate?

What a breathtaking entrance and lobby! Soaring ceilings with
long, sheer, flowing white drapes billowing in the ocean breeze, blur-
ring the definition between inside and out. There are walls but it
seems as if we are outside with the night air and fresh breeze blowing
through the hotel. All four walls of the dining room are lined with the
same gossamer white draperies, and all the beautiful waiters are
dressed from head to toe in white. The only decorations are etched
Venetian mirrors and a large mirrored pedestal in the center of the din-

ing room with a hundred ivory candles of different sizes and heights flickering in the gentle wind. It is so beautiful and elegant, a total thrill to the senses.

Dinner was sublime. I shared a salad of baby greens, pears, and prosciutto with mango–lime vinaigrette with Ronni. I had a tiny taste of a blue cheese Napoleon and of a crab–avocado terrine that were as delicious as they were beautiful. These plates of food were too much for words—each was an edible work of art. I ordered an entrée of lightly sautéed lobster on a crisp risotto cake with a passion fruit–herb reduction, braised baby bok choy, and cashews. It was very tender and really scrumptious. I was able to eat about half of the tail.

Dessert was going to be difficult, because they did not have any diabetic, sugar-free, or plain fruit desserts. I was going to have to implement the tiny taste method. Joyce had a Mango Baked Alaska, mango and passion fruit sorbet on an almond biscuit covered with meringue, baked and placed in the center of a huge pool of mango–passion fruit sauce with raspberry sauce swirls and chopped mangos. Not overly sweet, so I had two very small bites. Ronni had a melted chocolate cake with pistachio ice cream, one of those perfect little cakes that are hot liquid chocolate inside when you cut into it. I didn't taste that one at all because it looked too dangerously sweet. Another friend had a mascarpone cheesecake, a super-rich individual round with mango sauce on the plate and a burnt sugar crust. One small bite was divine. I also had a cappuccino with skim milk foam that was served in a beautiful oversized cup and saucer.

I'm thrilled that this surgery still allows me to do such great things and live life. Before my bariatric surgery, I was very worried that I would never be able to enjoy incredible evenings out, but it isn't a problem at all since there is always at least one good choice on any menu. I can't wait until I am even thinner in few months! I feel so healthy and strong and full of energy.

Tomorrow is part two of the birthday celebration. Ronni, Joyce, and I are spending the day at the Windham Bonaventure Spa. Six months ago I never would have considered something like this. I would have made excuses to avoid going. I am going to be one smooth and radiant chick when I get finished tomorrow.

November 5, 2001

Five years ago the owner of the company I was working with rewarded me with a full day at this same spa. I was humiliated within fifteen minutes of my arrival when the spa's robe didn't close and the staff acted as though no one had ever had this problem before. It was one of the worst days of my life. I spent every second not knowing whether to burst into tears or run out of there, but I had to stay since another manager had also been given the day off to use our motivational gift.

This time it was different. I was of normal size, comparatively speaking, and I wasn't embarrassed to disrobe alongside my slender friend Ronni in the women's locker room. She looked at me and couldn't believe how much smaller I was already. When I took the thick white terry robe off the hanger of my locker and slipped it on it was the moment of truth. The robe had plenty of overlap and felt soft and luxurious; I was so very happy.

We got our slippers and strolled into the salon for our pedicures. Next was my body treatment. When I walked into the wet treatment room and the clinician handed me a paper and elastic thong panty to put on—eeeeeeeeeeekkkkkkk! Scary to have to wear a thong—but it fit! I had to hang up my robe and lie face-down on the plastic-lined padded table while two clinicians with loofah mitts exfoliated the back of my body with the most delicious-smelling almond oatmeal scrub. My first thought was of how many carbs must be in the thick mixture! I had to flip over onto my back so they could scrub my front, and then flip over once again, no problem. Then they smoothed jet black Dead Sea mud all over me. I was wrapped in plastic sheets, then enveloped in thick heated padded blankets. The lights were dimmed and the women told me to relax for forty minutes. Wrapped in this warm cocoon, I thought about how different this spa trip was turning out; I gently fell in and out of a light sleep while I felt the warm mud squishing as I moved slightly. One woman unwrapped me while the other turned on the shower. When I stepped from the shower I was handed a towel for my hair which I fashioned into a turban and wrapped a second towel around me without thinking. Then it dawned on me that I just wrapped a towel around myself! Another thrilling moment and it wasn't even a large towel. I was glowing and not just from my mud treatment.

Now it was time for my facial. An older woman with a European accent came out and called my name. I followed her into the dimly lit room and reclined on the padded table. She put a bolster under my knees and a pillow under my head. A moist cloth was placed over my eyes and I was sprayed with a cool mist. My facial was incredible. She massaged the muscles in my neck and face and it felt so good I thought I was going to pass out.

I never dreamed in June that less than five months later I would actually have a great day at this spa. I started out a little nervous but left feeling soft and smooth and confident! I can't wait to go again.

November 27, 2001

We just returned home from Georgia after celebrating a Southern Thanksgivin' with my husband's kinfolk. As I had already anticipated, Georgia food was not good for me. The turkey was so overdone that it was like sawdust when you chewed it. Their family recipe for gravy involves cooking lard with flour and milk then adding chopped hardboiled eggs and chicken meat to the concoction. There was no way that I could moisten my food with this chunky slurry. I sneaked some of the drippings from the roasting pan into a cup and heated them in the microwave to pour over a few shreds of dark meat. I couldn't eat the sweet potato casserole made with brown sugar, marshmallows, and pecans. The vegetables were all cooked with fatback but they were at least tender, so I ate a few green beans. I couldn't eat the ham because it was too solid in consistency and dripping with cane syrup. It was a very difficult food day for me, and I ended up throwing up every bit that I ate. The only thing that was soft and easy for me to eat was the sugar-free pumpkin pie that I had baked at home and brought with us. To make it worse, everyone ate the leftovers for the next three days so I basically existed on my pie and coconut protein bars. I did wish that I could eat, but there will be other holidays when I will be able to prepare the food.

I felt so thin the entire time I was there and I knew I would lose a few pounds this Thanksgiving. Many of Ty's relatives didn't know how huge I was just five months ago and all they talked about was how pretty I was. It is hard to think of yourself as pretty when you were close to 300 pounds and you still have the fat clothes in your closet to remind you. I even asked Ty if the mirror in our bedroom was off and did it make him look thinner too. He laughed and said that the reflection was true and that I did look thin. When I weighed myself this morning I realized why I felt so thin; I am down to 180! I cannot believe it. I guess the plateau that had me bummed the last three weeks is over. The amazing part is that 4 pounds at this weight make a huge difference!

Ty's very petite and beautiful daughter Diane taught me a lesson about my changing body image. She weighs just 110 pounds and easily slips into a size 4, but her lower stomach is loose and stretched out after having three children. It made me very happy to see this! I don't mean that in a bad way because I love her dearly. We were talking about my weight loss and I told her about the embarrassing flap of skin squishing out over the waistband of my jeans, when she showed me her stomach. Seeing her belly and knowing how she felt made a big difference in how I feel about myself during this transitional weight-loss period. We women are all too tough on ourselves, no matter what our weight.

January 1, 2002

Wow . . . what a year for me! From a bursting-at-the-seams 278 to a still-shrinking 172 pounds in less than seven months. I never would have guessed it if you had asked me last January 1st, since I had not even thought about RNY surgery as a possibility at that point. I feel fantastic and I am gaining more confidence every day as I evolve.

My husband is giving me some trouble; he is having a hard time adjusting to the fact that I want to go out with my girlfriends to lunch and spend time doing things. I was essentially a shut-in by choice the last two years. I didn't get dressed up every day or do my hair or even put on makeup. I had such a low image of myself that I didn't care any more and made excuses to not take part in life. I talked to my girl-friends on the phone but didn't go anywhere with them. I hadn't stepped into a mall in over three years! Ty got used to this and since we work from home, he liked having me around 24/7. So now that his butterfly is flitting around and he's competing for my time, he is get-ting his back up. I am sure this has happened with many other women, and men, who have had this surgery. It may be amplified in my case, since my husband is twenty-two years older than I am. I met him when I was twenty-one but we have been together for almost twenty years. We have never had age issues and I don't think that this is necessarily the problem, but he keeps saying he knows how men are. I keep reminding him that I am not hanging out in bars and clubs, I am going to the mall or my girlfriends' houses. Things got a little tough around Christmas but seem better this week. I was spending a lot of time at Ronni's house baking cookies and gingerbread houses for Ty's grand-children. Now that the holidays are over I am sure that things will improve. Those of you who are married should prepare for changes in your spouse's attitude—it is inevitable. We have been together so long I just have to remind him that I am not going anywhere. Ty is a very exciting person to be with, always spontaneous and adventurous, and now that I am not dragging my feet and sabotaging his plans, we will enjoy many more years together.

February 8, 2002

The needle on the scale has not moved since Christmas. *This* is a plateau, not what people perceive as a plateau when they are ten weeks post-op. I am in my third week of a serious weight-lifting and aerobic exercise program, so I am fine with not having lost any more weight. I keep telling myself that just 12 months at 2 pounds a month will get me where I want to be. I am in perfect health.

Before I had my RNY surgery I had serious thyroid problems. In 1999 I had half of my thyroid removed when it was discovered that the gland was wrapped around my trachea and literally choking me. When it was removed, the surgeon found it had grown under my collarbone and into my chest cavity. Two weeks before my RNY surgery last June, my endocrinologist here in Fort Lauderdale wanted me to go off my Synthroid and have a nuclear test on a couple of nodules she spied on my latest thyroid ultrasound. If I went off my medicine, I would have been forced to cancel my gastric bypass surgery. After much thought, I decided that I would deal with my thyroid later and go ahead and have my RNY surgery. So now that I am eight months post-op gastric bypass surgery, I went ahead and scheduled a guided needle biopsy of those pesky nodules my endocrinologist wanted to have a look at. I was on the table; the ultrasound technician called in another technician, then another technician, and finally the radiologist. They were all taking turns on me with the rollerball probe to pinpoint what to biopsy before they inserted the needle. I was terrified, worrying about what they might have seen that was so devastating to keep all four gathered around the screen. They didn't see anything; there weren't any nodules. After losing all this weight and being on the same Synthroid dosage for these months, the nodules had disappeared! The radiologist was pleased to tell me that they couldn't locate any nodules in my neck to biopsy. The weight of the world was off my shoulders.

February 13, 2002

I have a girlfriend Stephanie, the same preoperative size as I was, who had her RNY procedure one week before I did. We were both unhappy about our clothes hanging from us as if they belonged to someone else, and decided to go on a shopping excursion to Macy's at Palm Beach Gardens Mall on Sunday. I do have to admit: it was one of my most inspired shopping trips to date. We had at least 100 pieces of clearance-priced clothing in those dressing rooms; then we swapped what didn't fit or what we didn't like by tossing it over the top of each other's booth, laughing the entire time. She is more of a 12 and I am a too-tight 12 and a better 14, so we are fairly compatible for shopping. Let me inquire though, just when was it decided that pants didn't need to come up past your belly button? I guess Lane Bryant didn't jump on *that* bandwagon. I had two epiphanies in that dressing room in a pair of size 12 DKNY pants as my loose belly fat spilled out and over the top of the incredibly low riding pants: first, that I didn't like this fashion trend at all and, second, that I am not as thin as I thought I was! The pants fit but it seemed like there were approximately four to six inches of vital fabric missing. Nope, the 14 didn't have any more coverage although they didn't seem to squeeze my Jell-O-like abdomen quite as obscenely. Hello fellow shoppers? Given that this *is* Palm Beach, would anyone in this dressing room have the number of a plastic surgeon handy?

We hit the food court and split a tuna wrap, picking apart our food like 4-year-olds, leaving the remains of our forage for protein on the tray. On the way past the Häagen-Dazs booth, Stephanie shared a bariatric secret with me. She asks for a sample of the Häagen-Dazs sugar-free soft yogurt and then savors the little free sample cup since she is now satisfied with just a taste. Not this time though. We shared a small cup of the creamy chocolate-vanilla swirl and I couldn't believe it wasn't full of sugar—it really tasted too good to be sugar-free. We sat on the edge of a planter and enjoyed our little treat.

Shopping is much better now than when I followed Ronni around the stores and suffered the embarrassment of leaving the dressing room to try to locate a size 2 from the rack before the genius salesgirls tracked me down to ask me what I was looking for. I always imagined they were laughing at me, thinking to themselves that nothing in the store would fit someone my size.

February 24, 2002

When you lose a lot of weight and get your life back, there are lots of crazy things you do that just a short time ago you would never even have thought of! My husband and I bought a Harley-Davidson V-Rod motorcycle two weeks ago and leased a condo on the ocean in Daytona Beach for Bike Week! I am amazed at how much fun my life is now—or maybe it just really sucked when I weighed almost 300 pounds. If you told me last year that I would be going to Daytona to party for Bike Week, I would have laughed at you. This is my first big adventure in at least two years, since we stopped vacationing when I was at my heaviest. I somehow squashed our sense of adventure by always making the dates inconvenient. I just manipulated our schedules in order to not get into uncomfortable situations on planes, in restaurants, amusement parks, rental cars, and boutiques with narrow aisles. I was hiding while life passed me by. I am ready to start living again and this time I am out of the chute on the back of a Harley! My family is beginning to worry about me.

March 9, 2002

We are home from Daytona and I had an amazing time! This was a week of fun, shiny chrome motorcycles, incredible people, and excellent food too! I can easily say that there was no way I could have ever done any of this without this surgery and losing all of that fat! I feel the urge to hug and kiss Dr. Carrasquilla right now. I didn't realize it, but our last few vacations were terrible. I felt so self-conscious about my appearance and tried so hard to avoid fat situations, that it made the trips into one-week-long arguments.

From day one I was perched on the back of that Harley looking cool in my black leather jacket and loving the attention that our motorcycle was getting and the attention that we were getting! I do have to say we had really great outfits. I love this biker thing as it combines a sport with fashion and makeup! I even bought a pair of black leather chaps; so now I am an official badass! The big joke among riders is the mystique of women wearing their chaps with just a thong. I really laughed at that one, as I definitely am not that kind of girl, but maybe I'll change my mind when I am 125 pounds.

We had a condo on this trip and I cooked big breakfasts for everyone each morning so I usually had an egg and some ham or sausage with a bite or two of biscuit. Lunch was a protein bar or some rolled up sandwich meat, and supper was shrimp or fish and a couple of raw oysters. I ate raw oysters all week; they were so good and easy to eat! I did have a few of what I would consider cheats during my week. I sampled a margarita that was made with fresh lime so there was no sugar or sweetened mix added. I drank half of that and got tipsy very quickly. I tasted a rum and Diet Coke and decided it was a horrible-tasting drink. I ate a few Fritos after my picnic lunch of a half turkey sandwich and threw everything up in the Kennedy Space Center parking lot. I had a few bites of the best Key Lime Pie I had ever tasted three nights in a row at an unbelievable fish camp restaurant. I had a spectacular time on this vacation and I even lost some weight. My butt felt smaller on that seat and my jeans are baggier because I managed to lose three pounds.

March 23, 2002

I am nine months, ten days post-op and we are going to a surprise birthday party for a friend tonight! No one from this group of friends has laid eyes on me since I was three months post-op and modeling my 1950s skirt and crinolines, so my weight loss didn't necessarily smack everyone in the face that night. I am sure everyone will notice my 117-pound loss tonight. The challenge is that the party is at Morton's of Chicago, home of very serious aged steaks. Most surgeons advise their patients to stay away from red meat for at least six months after surgery; it is often too difficult to digest. I really haven't missed it, but when we received the invitation, I started thinking about how good a few thin slices of filet mignon would taste.

Morton's is a very upscale steak house with dark wood paneling and a clubby feel to it, the kind of place with a cigar bar. Waiters fell over each other to keep a cocktail in your hand; huge silver platters of the biggest jumbo shrimp, absolutely enormous baked stuffed shrimp, tiny crab cakes, and baby lamb chops were carried around the room. The cocktail hour was not ending, and it looked like dinner was way off, so I decided to eat a shrimp and a crab cake. From 7:30 to 10:30 P.M. there was so much food I couldn't imagine how the rest of these folks were going to eat dinner. I drooled over the tiny lamb chops, but decided not to attempt that maneuver even though they looked very tender. One of our dear friends caught my eye from across the room and mouthed the words, "You look incredible, who are you?" Later on, when he made it across the room, he told me how perfect I looked. Then he back-pedaled, and said that I was always beautiful but NOW! It is funny when people catch themselves gushing over how great you look now but then don't want you to think they thought that you were a slug before you lost the weight. It meant a lot to me. I had been feeling a little fat—so many of the women were emaciated.

We weren't seated for dinner until almost 11:00. We had our choice of either a two-pound lobster out of the shell, twenty-ounce veal chop, or double filet mignon. Ty ordered the lobster and I ordered the filet but after an hour without the food appearing, I was thinking that I should have eaten a few more shrimp. Not that I was hungry, but I knew that I needed food. I was sipping some white wine and it went straight to my head, slurring my speech within minutes. It scared me and really freaked out my husband. He looked at me and asked me if I was all right and grabbed my hand, but I couldn't even answer him, my tongue was so thick. Then the feeling passed as quickly as it came over me and I felt a little dazed. They finally put my food in front of me at almost midnight. The filet had to weigh a pound! I sawed it in half and it was incredibly tender. This was an utterly fabulous piece of meat. I had to really concentrate on chewing it well. It actually made me a little sad that I could eat so little of it, but I just didn't have the room. By this time it was after 12:30, and all of us at the table were yawning while we ate. We decided to slip out before dessert without making a fuss. I wish I had the rest of that filet for tomorrow. Hell, I wish I had the rest of that filet to work on eating for the whole next week!

April 5, 2002

It is a glorious day here at the beach! The ocean is aqua and smooth. I am going to finish my protein shake and head out for a swim. Anyone who can't find a good tasting shake should try Zero Carb Isopure. The Creamy Vanilla is delicious when used as a base for creativity. I made a Cookies and Cream shake this morning to try something new and it tastes exactly like a Dairy Queen Blizzard. The key is to use a half cup of skim milk or water, 2 scoops of Isopure powder, and 1 cup of ice, and pulse the blender until the mixture is smooth and frosty. Then throw in 2 Murray's sugar-free chocolate cream-filled sandwich cookies and a tablespoon of Cool Whip and flip on the switch just long enough for the cookies to get sucked into the blades. It tastes amazing.

April 16, 2002

My grandmother will be 90 in May and my family has planned a party for her in New Jersey. This will be my first time on a plane since my surgery. Last night as I was choosing seats on the Expedia website, I had a flash of loathing for the middle seat and panicked about the flight. I never used a seatbelt extender, as I would rather have died during a free fall in turbulence than face the humiliation of publicly requesting one. I would suck in to snap the seatbelt, holding my breath until I passed the flight attendants' check, then quietly release the restraint without an audible click. I couldn't put my tray table down without it hitting my chest, so I had to say that I didn't want anything to eat or drink. Crowded flights were even more miserable, with my poor husband having to endure my being jammed into his side for hours so I didn't take up any of the window passengers' space. I can imagine how awful flying is for people who are even larger than I was. And of course, five out of ten times I would have a "recliner" in front of me. I would tap on the back of their seat, firmly telling them that with seats as close as they are on planes, there just wasn't enough room with their seat back, and could they please put it up. I know that even when I am thin, I will not recline on planes, knowing how uncomfortable it makes larger people who don't have the voice to say anything.

May 1, 2002

I am discovering that I can eat slightly larger quantities of food than I could initially, and that it would be easy to eat the wrong foods. I notice that some of the others who had their surgery about the same time as I did are really off track with the food choices they are making and the amount of sugar they know they can tolerate. My surgery was almost eleven months ago and I am not done losing weight yet; I don't want to eat anything that will slow down my loss or prevent me from getting to my goal weight. There are women from my surgical support group who talk about eating at Taco Bell or Wendy's, and how much of a Subway sandwich they can consume. They laugh nervously about eating mini-Snickers bars and how regular ice cream doesn't make them "dump." They eat baked potatoes, bread, rolls, and crackers, and think nothing of it because they are still limited in their volume. To me, every bite of carbohydrate prevents me from burning my stored fat. I have taken a completely different approach to using my pouch as a tool for life. I didn't enter into this process thinking that I would only have to change my diet for a few months and then could go back to eating the same way I did before my surgery. I made a resolution that I would change the way I made decisions about food and would make these changes permanent to my lifestyle. I just don't cook foods that don't work for my dietary requirements; I watch every gram of carbohydrate that I eat, and rarely buy bread or crackers anymore. There are times when I need something crunchy with my shrimp salad; but if I am going to eat a few crackers, I count them out and make sure that I compensate by having fewer carbohydrates for supper. I don't feel sad that I can't eat the entire box of Cheez-Its, I am thankful that I can eat ten of them while wearing size 12 jeans. Many people who have bariatric surgery don't realize that they have a seven- to ten-month window of opportunity to maximize their weight loss, and after that time the rate of loss declines drastically.

May 21, 2002

Grandma's birthday bash was wonderful and she never looked younger or more beautiful! I am so thankful for good genes, even if some of them are fat genes. Her skin is flawless, and her neck and chest aren't wrinkled at all. She is the epitome of classic Italian beauty— snow-white hair and sparkling hazel eyes with a touch of mischief in them—and still sharp as a razor and spry as a 40-year-old. When she realized that this was no ordinary birthday dinner she laughed, then cried tears of joy as she realized all her family had gathered to celebrate her 90 years of life. It was an incredible day and Grandma Helen proclaimed it the greatest day of her life. As she blew out the candles on her Italian cream cake she asked God for ten more years. I am sure he is working on it right now.

When she found out we were all taking her to Atlantic City in the morning, nothing else mattered for the evening. The next day we arrived to pick her up and she had prepared the Italian Grandma Special of manicotti, meatballs, and tossed salad. It was delicious and we all laughed as Grandma kept telling me to eat more food. When we arrived at the casino, Grandma practically ran through the lobby toward the slot machines, and walked up and down the aisles until she found the one she felt was ready to pay off. We knew where she would be for the next few hours, so we decided to find a blackjack table. I moved through the casino feeling great about myself, feeling light, feeling beautiful, feeling small, finally rid of the baggage I carried for so many years. We played blackjack for six hours straight and our little pile of green chips grew to several piles of black chips—we were almost $3000 ahead by suppertime. It was time to retrieve Grandma and the rest of the family, and since we were the big winners it would be our treat at the casino's gourmet seafood restaurant. However, Grandma had beat us to it: she had gone to the host window and cashed in her "comps" to take all of us to dinner at the buffet. I couldn't eat the featured prime rib—it was too dense and dry—but she was so proud to take us all to dinner on her winnings that it didn't matter at all.

June 1, 2002

Just ten days to go to celebrate my one-year surgery date! I am leaving in two days on a trip to Germany with my brother, John. He works for Mercedes-Benz and one of his clients wanted a special edition car that has a lengthy waiting list in the U.S. The only way for this man to get his hands on one of these cars is to take delivery in Europe under a special program. The Mercedes-Benz factory keeps a few of the really special cars such as the CL55 AMG for this select program, but this client really had no intention of going to Germany to get it. Yep, he plotted to send my brother, but didn't tell him until after he had ordered the car. So my brother has to pick up this incredible car from the factory in Stuttgart and enjoy the royal treatment that Mercedes-Benz lavishes on clients buying $115,000 cars. How do I fit into this picture? John's wife would never leave their 3-year-old son, Alec, with anyone, not even to go to the store or the mall, and she surely wouldn't leave him for a week while she goes to Germany with my brother. So, I told John that I would go with him! I fly out of Miami, he flies from Newark, we meet in London, then fly together to Stuttgart, Germany. I am so excited—I have never been to Europe before. My brother won't be driving the client's new car while we are in Germany; as much as he would love to take this mega-fast AMG car out on the autobahn, a scratch would mean curtains for his job, so John will sign for it and take it to the parking lot on the other side of the factory, where it will be shipped to New Jersey. Then we rent our own smaller Benz and are off on our Black Forest rally. I didn't know anything about this area, but now that I have checked it out on the Internet, I know it is going to be fabulous. Of course I researched and found the name of the place that reportedly has the best Black Forest Cake on the planet and learned how to say it in German even though I can only savor three bites of *Schwarzwalder Kirschtorte!* I told John to smack the fork from my hand if I go for a fourth bite or he would be carrying me out of the place. The area is also known for its handmade sausages and cured hams. I am packing plenty of protein bars and two packs of EAS AdvantEdge Carb Control chocolate premixed drinks just in case I can't eat.

I decided that on the way home, instead of just changing planes at Heathrow, I would stay a night in London to celebrate my one-year anniversary date. My brother has to continue on home, but being alone is not a bad thing. I am celebrating my newfound strength and life. While I would love to be with my husband, this time alone is not so bad. I am going to check into the Connaught, one of London's finest hotels. I can't wait to go to dinner at the finest restaurant in London and raise my glass in a toast "to Susan." I am pissed that Paul McCartney is getting married this week. I am a week too late to win the heart of my favorite Beatle. Celebrating my one-year birthday at 149 pounds in London is going to be the best part. I will drink in all the flavors and take in the sites and have a great trip. Life just gets better and better all the time as I get smaller and smaller! Paul's loss.

June 11, 2002

One year ago yesterday I began my new life. I cannot believe this past year and how much has changed for me. I returned from the most fabulous trip of my life late last night and none of it would have happened without my surgery last June.

I am 147 pounds this morning, so I have lost 131 pounds in this very full and remarkable year. I should be winding down with losing but I am sure that I will continue to slowly lose over the next few months, which is fine with me. The size 10 BCBG jeans I bought for my trip were a little big yesterday so I am sure 8s are coming by next month. I dwell on how I look sometimes because it is amazing to look in the mirror and see someone you don't recognize as you, but I walked for miles around Germany and London with extra energy and climbed mountains of stairs and could have gone on forever. That is what this procedure is all about: health and fitness. The fact that I regained lost beauty and youth is a gift!

Germany was incredible; the country is simply the most beautiful place I have ever been. Picking up John's client's car was a blast; we had a tour of the Mercedes-Benz factory and were treated to a gourmet dinner in their elegant restaurant. White asparagus are in peak season at the moment, and all the restaurants in this area celebrate the greatly anticipated, short season by having a *Spargelkart*, or Asparagus menu, with 4- and 5-course dinners that feature these delicate rarities as the star. So my "foodie" brother and I dove right in and had cream of asparagus soup, asparagus salad, and asparagus with hollandaise and prawns as the main course, a large pile of tender logs of white asparagus napped with the delicious classic lemon butter sauce. The prawns were there as an afterthought, as the asparagus were the centerpiece of this amazing dish. I had never tasted fresh white asparagus before but they were incredible with a very delicate flavor. I sliced the thick spears into thin slices and with the sauce had no trouble eating about half of my pile of ten spears.

The hotels that Mercedes-Benz chooses for the Euro delivery clients are amazing. To say that the *Schlosshotel Buhlerhohe* was luxurious is an understatement, a grand hotel and spa built at the turn of the twentieth century that has been completely and magnificently restored. The views are breathtaking, taking in miles of mountains with the Swiss Alps in the distance. We were treated like royalty with an international array of polite and crisp waiters and butlers catering to our every whim. A wonderful European custom is to have a late afternoon snack of tea or coffee and pastry. We had cafe macchiatos and I selected a rhubarb cream torte from the pastry cart. It had a buttery shortbread crust, a thick layer of tangy buttermilk or yogurt custard topped with tart sliced rhubarb; not a sweet pastry by any means, but as it was definitely not sugar-free I gathered up all my willpower and ate a little less than half of the large slice, not wanting to test my dumping mechanism in the middle of this grand drawing room. It was heavenly and I found that I have a very good handle on my willpower when it is backed by fear. My brother had his first of many large hunks of Black Forest Cake—German chocolate cake layered with whipped cream and cherries soaked in the local cherry liqueur. The bite I sampled was ethereal.

We spent the afternoon exploring the area and had a late dinner in our hotel's celebrated restaurant. The rain had started to fall and our views were now of the milky white clouds that obscured our earlier panorama. Dinner was fabulous but my brother still could not get over the fact that my plate is always less than half eaten. He did comment though that I was not a cheap date, since I still order the same plate of food; I am a *wasteful* date. I ordered a coffee crème brûlée for dessert; it was silky and cold with the hot crisp caramelized sugar crust on top, served with a plate of fresh plum compote and a platter of petit fours that were miniature works of art! John didn't want dessert but once this extravagance was put in front of me and I only ate 3 spoonfuls of the crème brûlée, he picked up the spoon and finished off all the sweet treats, mumbling what a waste it would be to not eat this incredible food.

After one year, dumping syndrome is still a very real fear to me. I have not tested my limits; in fact I am careful not to cross my self-imposed line of five to eight grams of sugar at one time. I don't feel deprived, rather I feel blessed that I can enjoy a formal or gourmet meal including an incredible dessert and stay within my boundaries of carbohydrates and sugar. This surgical procedure has given me strength, and is a tool that allows me to taste but not overeat. I have friends who have tested their sugar limits and are distraught that they "do not dump," thereby giving them permission to step out of the RNY limits and cheat. I am convinced that these folks will regain some of their weight and have a harder time maintaining long-term weight loss even with the surgical limitations of their stomach volume. I have to be satisfied with a taste of dessert backed with the fear of dumping. Later that night, I kept repeating this to myself in order to keep my hand from stuffing the handmade chocolates that I found on my night-stand directly into my mouth.

Our flight touched down in London and I tearfully said goodbye to my wonderful brother at Heathrow airport. John and I have cooked together and talked food for years and there is no one I know of in this world who could have been as perfectly paired with him to share this epicurean journey. I grabbed the London express train and within a half hour of landing at Heathrow was sitting by myself in the magnificent lobby of my London hotel. The Connaught is old money, old world, old attitude, and incredibly stuffy; I loved it. Would Madame like a pot of tea while the bellman takes her bags up to her room and her butler unpacks for her? Absolutely! I thought of my mother and that I knew she was watching over me and smiling while I enjoyed my moment of extreme sophistication.

I finished my tea then climbed the staircase up to my room where my mind was immediately blown! The room was just lovely with fabrics in bright yellows, greens, and touches of burgundy, a Louis XIV writing desk, a goose down comforter and linen duvet, eight linen-covered down pillows piled against the headboard, a magnificent green Murano glass chandelier hanging from the ceiling, a massive antique mahogany wardrobe, a thick Frette terry robe to luxuriate in, and a marble bath with shining silver fixtures. I changed my clothes and headed out to explore London.

I am writing all this in such detail because just a year ago I would have never done any of it! I wouldn't have had the guts to get on a plane and head off to Germany, never mind be in London by myself. As a fat girl I was too self-conscious, always thinking people were looking at me and judging me, laughing at me. Maybe they were, and maybe they weren't, but it sure stopped me from living. The new me is free and bold, as I love life and myself. So don't think that I am getting too far off topic. While in London I feel tall, I feel thin, and I feel beautiful.

I bought a ticket and boarded a double-decker bus. I was the only patron and as I climbed the narrow metal spiral staircase to the top deck the reality struck me that not too many months ago I was too large to fit. Perched high atop the moving bus I had a wonderful vantage point for all of London's sights and a personal tour guide to explain everything I was seeing. I had a great afternoon with James, my tour guide, even when the inevitable London rain commenced. After the tour, I said goodbye to James and my bus driver, and walked back to the hotel with my mascara streaming down my face, looking a bit like Ozzie Osborne, my hair in soaked ringlets around my face. I was miserably wet. The doorman recognized my pitiful condition and suggested that I have some hot tea in the drawing room. That sounded good to me. I sat down and in minutes the formal white-gloved waiter placed a silver tea service in front of me. There were 6 kinds of sugar—brown rock crystals, white rock crystals, brown cubes, white cubes, brown granules, white granules, but just one kind of sugar substitute: an envelope with two tiny white saccharin pills. I drank it plain, just a touch of cream, rather than taint it with saccharin. The concierge came over and asked me if Madame would like him to have my butler draw me a hot bath while Madame drinks her tea? After her tea, Madame had a hot bath and when she was done the sun was shining, so Madame dried off, did her makeup and hair, got dressed, this time grabbing an umbrella from the concierge and was off on round two of her adventure! Walk, walk, walk, walk, walk, walk, walk, walk, walk, walk, walk, walk—wow, what energy I have at 147 pounds! The 300-pound Susan would have stayed in the hotel—actually the 300-pound Susan would be sitting at home in Florida. I had a bounce in my step and all the confidence in the world as I made my way around this gorgeous city.

I glanced at my watch, I couldn't believe how time had quickly passed and it was time for the appointment that I made for the London Eye. The British Airways Millennium Wheel is a 50-story, constantly moving observation wheel with 25 giant glass pods that allow amazing views over the city of London and the countryside. I quickly located it in the skyline and ran so I wouldn't miss my reservation. I was upset that I had arrived ten minutes after my time slot. But when I swiped my Visa in the machine to retrieve my ticket, out popped the ticket. I stood on the platform and thought about times I dreaded stepping onto an elevator because of the embarrassing lurch my weight would cause—and here I was ready to step into a huge glass egg without hesitation. A beautiful family from India and a local London family who pointed out the sites were my mates for this trip as we ascended to almost 500 feet in the sky. What an incredible feeling of freedom. It was almost 9:00 P.M. yet the stone buildings of London were reflecting the glow of the bright orange late-afternoon sun as we slowly rotated around the giant spoked wheel. It was simply breathtaking.

The Connaught has a Michelin-starred restaurant and since I was alone, I thought it best to eat in the hotel rather than wander London after dark. I dashed upstairs and fluffed my hair, jazzed up my makeup, stopped for a minute to celebrate the fact that I could now wear size B pantyhose, slipped on a slinky black T dress, slid into my high heels, wrapped my new French blue cashmere pashmina around my shoulders and added blue topaz and diamond earrings and bracelets. I felt like Princess Diana as I descended the stairs to the lobby. The maître d' welcomed me, seated me facing the room at a lovely table and I suddenly had all eyes of the room upon me. I sipped my Kir Royale—champagne with just a drop of Chambord liqueur—and softly smiled while I studied the menu for easy-to-eat choices in one of the world's finest restaurants. I decided on the terrine of foie gras as an appetizer and the roasted Dover sole served with an English mustard-butter sauce and sautéed baby spinach. The terrine was incredible, but I ate just half of the thin slice knowing that room in my pouch was limited. I ignored the breadbasket on my table, though with great difficulty. The Dover sole was presented in an enormous silver domed platter and set atop a silver frame while the waiter expertly deboned the whole roasted fish and plated it, spooning on a creamy mustard sauce. I ate about half of the moist, perfectly cooked and seasoned fish along with a few bites of the sautéed spinach before I became very full. I sipped a crisp Chardonnay along with my fish, selected by the sommelier to go with my sole. I never drink with my meals but this was the exception. The waiters fell over themselves to take care of me and keep me entertained. After my meal, the headwaiter tempted me with the dessert cart and after I explained I had to choose a less-sugared dessert because I was a "diabetic," we discussed the merits of each of the desserts on the cart. He could have the dessert chef prepare a simple compote of stewed, unsweetened fresh fruits as there were bowls of poached apricots, pitted cherries, strawberries, rhubarb, and pears; or I could choose a decadent and fabulous sugary creation knowing I couldn't risk a fourth bite. John had convinced me that a tiny taste of something spectacular was better than a whole lot of something ordinary. I chose a Spring Cup, a beautifully etched martini glass with thin, even layers of pistachio mousse, dense, tart apricot puree, bittersweet chocolate mousse, milk chocolate mousse, and vanilla-bean cream. The colors in this dessert were so soft and beautiful that if its stripes were of silk it would be my favorite scarf. It was a work of art and I precisely measured out a reasonable amount of this unreasonable dessert on my spoon and slowly let it dissolve in my mouth. The flavors were incredible and intense. After savoring a safe amount, I pushed the plate to the far side of the table and it was quickly whisked away. I smiled as I climbed the winding dark wood staircase to my room. The butler had turned down my bed and the fine linens felt so soft and wonderful. I thought about my spectacular day in London and fell into a deep sleep. For the first time in many years I was confident that there was no way that my dreams could possibly surpass the reality of this last week.

July 22, 2002

My husband and I were having dinner at the Fifth Avenue Grill on Friday evening, a celebration dinner of sorts for a couple of big deals we closed earlier that day, when I casually suggested that we should go to Las Vegas this weekend. Or maybe it was my husband who said it first, I really don't recall. Maybe it was his Beefeater Martini or possibly my Peppar Bloody Mary that made it seem like a great suggestion, but we both jumped on it. When we got home I logged onto Orbitz.com, found two nonstop tickets to Las Vegas, threw a few things in our bags, and we headed to the airport. A tuxedoed driver in his silver limousine met us, compliments of the Mirage, and within six hours of our dinner, we were checking in at the VIP office of one of the most exciting places in the world.

It was 2:00 A.M. Las Vegas time, and the Mirage was as beautiful as I remembered. We took the private elevator to our floor, quickly unpacked, regrouped and were at a blackjack table in twenty minutes, playing cards and having a ball until dawn. We staggered upstairs and got a couple of hours sleep courtesy of the room darkening shades before my ultimate bariatric test: the Mirage brunch buffet. I used to dream about this buffet; my husband used to tease me about having prime rib for breakfast in my old life. I was hesitant about standing in front of the largest food orgy in Las Vegas and trying to select a few bites of protein, but I was up for the challenge. Was the quality as good as the quantity or was the sheer volume what I loved about this buffet in the past? I grabbed a large plate and decided on some chilled jumbo shrimp, a cheese blintz, and a few slices of smoked salmon to roll up with cream cheese, red onion, and capers. It was hard not to let my eyes be too much bigger than my stomach. It is tough to take one of something small, but I am learning. Everything was delicious and I didn't miss the mountains of food on my plate at all. Sitting there in size 10 jeans was no doubt a factor. Food no longer rules me, but I still went back to the dessert buffet and got a tiny espresso cup of crème brûlée to satisfy my love for the stuff and had my obligatory spoonful. I was stuffed and overjoyed.

Back at the blackjack tables, we spent hours attempting to break the house. All day long we were up and down, never quite reaching my husband's goal in order to quit winners. We had a blast and laughed as we did twenty years ago when he first brought me to Las Vegas.

During a break from the tables we strolled past the jewelry shop to look at watches and I spied a gorgeous David Yurman ring that matched a bracelet I had bought there with blackjack winnings eight years ago. I have lost so much weight that all my rings fall off my fingers and seem too large in style for my now more-petite hands. Even my diamond wedding band needs to be completely remade, as the thick, size 10½ pavé band is ridiculously large. The ring in the case was a gorgeous gold and silver twisted band featuring a large, faceted peridot stone. I left the store with the ring and the matching earrings. Life is cool.

The next twenty-four hours was a blur of blackjack, a romantic lobster tail dinner in the middle of the Mirage rainforest, a great show, and more blackjack. We caught our limo at the north entrance of the hotel and were deposited at the airport at 11:00 P.M. for our red-eye flight home to Miami. We walked in the door of our condo at 9:00 A.M. yesterday morning and I sit here laughing about our whirlwind black-jack tour of the Mirage. Only the dazzling ring on my finger confirms our last two days of spontaneity and laughter!

September 2, 2002

I celebrated my forty-first birthday on August 30th. I wasn't upset about it, though. I was upset on my fortieth birthday because I was so huge and joked at the time that forty-one and thin would be much better than forty and fat. It is true! Being forty-one years old is extraordinary. We celebrated with dinner at Morton's, and I wore the magnificent blouse I bought at a boutique in the Mirage Shops in Vegas. It is all leopard and lace print in browns, black and white, shredded, crinkled, and see-through, it wraps around my body and ties, major cleavage, the sleeves are long and uneven, it is so cool and sexy, I love it! Ty looked pretty good too—he is a striking man and we really look good together again. I had a Peppar Bloody Mary and he had a Beefeater Martini, along with some tiny west coast oysters, of which I ate two. I ordered filet Oscar, a seared filet mignon, butterflied and topped with lump crabmeat and perfect hollandaise sauce. Ty, being a fish-eating vegetarian, ordered crab cakes. The filet was fork tender; I ate almost one half of the moist, crab-topped steak before I was very full. We lingered and the waiter brought over the dessert tray. We decided on cappuccino and I chose the cheesecake. My husband wanted me to choose key lime pie. I told him that it is too much sugar and that I wanted a bite of cheesecake. He made a face and said he wants me to get the pie, as in his opinion key lime pie is better than cheesecake. I pulled rank and firmly told him that he doesn't get to choose, since it is *my* birthday! So I have now inadvertently informed the waiter that it is my birthday. Thanks a lot, Ty, now I had candles on my cheesecake as it crossed the room, but at least the waiters didn't sing to me. The upshot was that I won and got a bite of cheesecake, plus it was on the house. It was a fun evening and we strolled hand in hand from the restaurant even after the ugly cheesecake incident.

September 12, 2002

It is miraculous how even the way you think about food changes during the months after your surgery. Now that I am fifteen months post-op I suddenly feel so normal about eating small portions. I really enjoy good food even with a stomach the size of a small lemon. I savor the food and take pleasure in the flavors. I eat slowly, actually putting my fork down while chewing and tasting, instead of finishing my entire plate in minutes. When I look at the menu I select something that appeals to me rather than thinking about the portion size. I don't worry that the crab appetizer I order for my entrée will be small. I weigh the value of each morsel and prioritize what I want to put into my mouth, eating the best bites first. I think about what I really want and what will work for me, it isn't a mindless overindulgence anymore. I cannot believe how my entire relationship with food has changed.

My sudden weight loss has left me with an unsightly flap of skin hanging from my lower belly called a panniculus. The surgical procedure in which this skin is removed, called a panniculectomy, is usually performed in tandem with a tightening of the underlying abdominal muscles, or abdominoplasty. I had a consultation with a plastic surgeon on Tuesday and scheduled my reconstructive surgery. I really like the no-nonsense approach of the surgeon, and the fact that he was a professor at Duke University Medical School. Dr. Rainer Sachse performed a hernia operation, surgical scar revision, and tummy tuck on my girlfriend Dhona; her scar is amazingly thin and well hidden, and her stomach is completely flat and taut. He was very confident that he could remove all of the excess belly fat and skin from my stomach using a slightly extended version of the regular abdominoplasty scar going about six inches past each of my hipbones. I am very fortunate that my arms and legs are small, with little excess skin; all my extra weight is in my lower stomach. I can actually grab it with my hands and pull it away from my abdomen similar to what the surgeon will be doing with this operation. I will be so small when those 8 pounds of fat and skin are gone. It is frightening to me to go under general anesthesia again, but I cannot imagine going through all this and not completing the last few yards. I don't think that I need the abdominoplasty procedure but I do want it. The date is set for October 24, 2002. All the surgeons I interviewed said that there is no way insurance will cover a dime of the procedure because my skin flap doesn't even lap over, so I will have to pay for it myself.

I have been going through the emotions of my gastric bypass surgery again as my girlfriend Jo had her laparoscopic RNY surgery last Thursday; she is one week post-op today and is doing absolutely fantastically. She spent just two nights in the hospital and was feeling pretty funky the first night, but after that there was no stopping her from walking up and down those halls. Her surgeon is a little different with his initial food requirements in that she is to stick to clear liquids for an additional week, so I made a pot of homemade chicken broth today to take to her house in the morning. When I was one week post-op I was still sitting in my hospital bed sucking on ice chips but when I returned home I really appreciated a steaming mug of homemade chicken broth—it was so soothing and warm going down. Jo is 66, a retired special education teacher who lives next door to my Dad. She watched in awe as I melted before her eyes over the last year. She shocked all of us when she announced that she was going to have the surgery. Many of her friends tried to talk her out of it, telling her she was too old. She weighed the positives and negatives and made her decision based on the facts as they pertained to her. Jo decided that she was 66 years young, not old, and that she was heading down a rough road weighing 235 pounds at a mere 4 feet, 10 inches. She is already telling the naysayers that "nothing tastes as good as thin feels" when they ask her if she misses eating. She is a good student and she is going to be so cute when she is little. She reminds me quite frequently that she is the same height as Judy Garland, and is such a great lady. Her blood pressure has already dropped to normal levels, her cholesterol has plummeted, and she is full of energy.

October 5, 2002

We went on the annual Harley-Davidson Key West Poker Run with some of our yuppie biker friends. What fun! You leave Miami and while en route to Key West you make five designated stops, choosing a playing card from a deck of cards at each stop. At the last stop the person with the best poker hand wins either cash or a new Harley. There were over 10,000 motorcycles participating, even with Hurricane Isadore swirling in the gulf. From the back of the V-Rod I enjoyed the perfect vantage point to watch hundreds of motorcycles cruising over the seven-mile bridge in Marathon Key with the turquoise water, and palm trees swaying in the background. Life was a postcard! Downtown was packed and I got to be a bad biker mama for the weekend. Two of the wives asked me why I didn't just let go and splurge for a special occasion. They had noticed how careful I am about what I eat. I just reiterated that I didn't like to be overstuffed when I was on the motorcycle and left it at that. I feel guilty that they admire my control. If they only knew.

When we got home I discovered that my friend Jo had been hospitalized! Apparently she didn't think that water was important and she wasn't drinking any. She also wasn't eating enough food and didn't want to drink the protein shakes I told her she should be sipping. She was taken to the emergency room while we were in Key West and they threw her in a bed with two IVs for severe dehydration. So with Ty in bed at home, sick with bronchitis, I left him to go to the hospital every day because Jo was a total wreck, crying and whimpering. She was scared to death she was dying. I needed to hold her hand and keep telling her that she didn't have anything wrong with her that would kill her, but if she didn't start drinking water, I would kill her. After eleven days, she is home and has learned that food and water are important after weight-loss surgery. If you are having a problem that prevents you from eating or drinking, you have to call your surgeon's office. Jo cannot cook to save her life, so once I took her home I went to the store and bought some cooked shrimp, turkey breast, cheese, cottage cheese, and some of the EAS Carb Control premixed chocolate protein shakes. I chopped the cooked shrimp and blended them with a couple of spoonfuls of low sugar cocktail sauce so it would be moist, and put the bowl in her refrigerator. I cooked some sugar-free chocolate pudding and whisked in a couple of scoops of protein powder. I instructed her to eat little portions, make sure she waits an hour after eating before drinking, and other than that she needed to sip water constantly while walking. This time she is going to be fine. I am not sure she knew that it wasn't all cake and roses from 278 pounds to where I am now. It takes dedication to health, and you must follow the rules of eating and, just as important, drinking. Sixty-four ounces of water doesn't seem like a lot until you are on your third eight-ounce glass of the day, which you are managing to funnel through a very small opening.

October 22, 2002

While we were on a weekend trip to Daytona Beach on our Harley, we decided to head over to Universal Studios in Orlando for the day. We had a light breakfast and were pulling through the Universal Studio's gates in about an hour. We practically ran through the gates of Islands of Adventures and stopped short to gaze at the incredible roller coasters. I hadn't been on a ride in years. I would never admit that it was because of my weight, but now I am certain that I was afraid of not fitting on the rides. I know people who had to face the humiliation of not being able to fit in the seat, or being too large for the restraint device to lock. I stared at the Incredible Hulk roller coaster and had to try it. As the hydraulic bar locked into place over my body, I was secretly relieved that it fit. It was an irrational fear but my heart still raced. I started screaming from the moment I was first turned upside-down and didn't stop until my feet were back on the ground. I can't believe I had convinced myself I didn't like this kind of ride. On to Fire and Ice Dueling Dragons, two separate roller coasters that intertwine; when you are on Fire, your body is flying mere inches away from the people who are riding on Ice. We decided to have a snack as Ty spied a candy shop. There were huge bins of sugar-free Jelly Belly beans in delicious flavors and I filled a bag with almost a pound of the intensely fruity candies. I placed the open bag in my leather Harley pouch and started munching on them as we walked through the rest of the park. While we were considering our next roller coaster ride I felt the unmistakable rumble of my stomach telling me that I was getting ready to have an immediate and severe problem. I had eaten almost half of the sugar-free candy, which doesn't affect blood sugar levels because maltitol sweetener isn't absorbed in the intestines. However, there are warnings on foods containing maltitol and I was about to have a lesson confirming why this is so. It was very stupid to eat that much sugar-free candy and after a brief restroom tour of the park, I was ready to leave.

October 27, 2002

It is less than three days since I went in for my plastic surgery procedure and I feel terrific! I have felt wonderful since the moment I opened my eyes after my surgery. I never experienced that horrible, groggy, heavy headache feeling from the anesthesia. This anesthesiologist must have done something different. I felt awful when I woke up from my other two surgeries, but this one was like waking up from a nap. I had no pain to speak of, just a fear of moving! I started to get a bit nauseous and the nurse put an alcohol pad to my nose and the feeling went away immediately. Nice trick. They helped me up from the bed and walked me over to a recliner chair. I put on my sweatpants and zippered sweatshirt and felt great. I was moving slowly but it was from the thick bandages and drains hanging from the bandages. I cannot stand up straight and have to walk hunched over. I decided that my own bed would be a wonderful thing and soon I was in a wheelchair heading toward my car. My sweet husband had brought a pillow for me to hug, but I really didn't need it. I was alert but a little foggy now and then. I don't remember the trip, but I did get nauseous in our elevator and had to spit up just as I was walking to my bedroom. Poor Ty was walking with all my stuff and didn't know what I needed, and of course my mouth was full of spit. I just stood there looking at the little pink dish he was holding. I finally snatched it from him and then remembered that I had an alcohol pad in my pocket that the nurse gave me just in case. It worked in time and I didn't throw up. Minor tragedy averted, as I am sure that throwing up would have hurt. Ty fixed my pillows so that I could sit up against the headboard. He had at least eight pillows for me, and propped up my legs and arms so I was comfy. I dozed off for a few hours but then woke with great clarity and can honestly say that I felt so much better than I had anticipated. I took several naps and started on my pain pills and antibiotics, making sure I ate a cracker with each pill to avoid nausea.

When I am in bed and look down at myself, it is like gazing at someone else's body. I don't recognize my own torso; it looks nothing like anything I have seen for the past 40 years. When the bandages are removed, I have a nice new deep belly button, a wide expanse of flat belly, and my abdomen flows neatly into my narrow hips. Granted, I look as if I have been nearly severed in half, but I'm not all bruised and swollen as I thought I would be. This is simply amazing. On June 10,

2001, I was 278 pounds and miserable, and this morning, except for the stitches, I am happy and look like I could be in a magazine. A shower can only improve things.

November 4, 2002

This is Day 11 post-op abdominoplasty and my drains are still in. Once I get them out I will be 100 percent back to normal within a day or two. I am sure that my body is fighting the intrusion of the couple of feet of plastic tubing, draining me of energy. I have been out of the house a couple of times but I am just too worried that I will rip out a tube by catching it on something, so my excursions have been limited. The incision is perfect except for a one-inch segment that looks a bit rough. I have only a few very faint bruises and my new belly button is a very attractive, vertically-oriented little oval! My stitches are on the inside, no staples or black thread, just a perfectly, smoothly matched incision where the skin comes together. I have some swelling but already I have a nice smooth line now that I have switched to a high-waisted elastic panty garment. This surgery has gone perfectly for me. My friend Stephanie has had her tummy tuck as well. Her surgeon was apparently too aggressive and may have removed too much tissue and stretched her skin too tightly, compromising the blood supply between her new belly button and incision. This is called *tissue necrosis* and I don't think that she understands that she is going to have a lengthy recovery. I do believe that her wound is going to get much worse before it gets better, and this will be incredibly traumatic for her. Once again I am incredibly thankful for my excellent surgeon.

November 19, 2002

I am now four weeks post-op abdominoplasty and I feel fantastic! Drains are out, the incision is a faint pink line, and I have very little swelling remaining. I have a perfectly flat stomach! I can finally fit into my pre-op clothes, and they are big in the area below the waistband. They fit in the waist but there is this big baggy area where I used to have all the belly flab. I stare at myself in the mirror all the time; I can't believe that I am this thin. Now that the swelling has subsided, I can wear any size 8 and actually fit into some size 6 skirts and pants. My mind is totally blown! When I had the weight loss surgery I set my goal conservatively at a size 12 and decided that if I didn't get any smaller than that I would still be thrilled. I can't even imagine wearing a size 6. I don't feel that small and in fact I still judge the spaces where I need to walk. I thought about it the other day when I got up from a restaurant table and went around the long way to avoid having to squeeze between chairs even though there was plenty of room. I was making my calculations based on the 278-pound body size instead of my new smaller mass. I wonder if I will ever feel small without looking in a mirror.

For the first time since having my weight loss surgery, I experienced "dumping syndrome" from too much sugar while I was visiting Ty's family in Georgia. I have been so careful to avoid it over the past eighteen months. We were celebrating Uncle Billy's birthday at the farm and his daughter Barbara had baked a cake for him. I ate one layer of a thin slice of the cake, somehow completely misjudging the sugar grams that I was ingesting. Within minutes, I began to sweat profusely and got very dizzy. I asked Ty to take me outside so I could walk around in the cold fresh air, but then I had to come right back in and sit down on the sofa. I was hoping to avoid a scene and just stay in the living room while everyone finished their dessert. Then my stomach and intestines started to seize up inside of me and I had horrible abdominal pain. I thought I was going to die and unfortunately all of my in-laws thought so, too. Everyone gathered around me and kept asking me if I was all right. I was in absolute agony for about twenty minutes and didn't move for lack of knowing what the hell I was going to do. When I would breathe I would feel a sharp, stabbing pain in the area of my stomach pouch and intestines so I took shallow gulps of air.

Then as fast as it came over me, it subsided and I was perfectly fine. I will be so much more careful from now on. I knew I shouldn't have had that last bite or two of cake. I am very upset that I did this to myself, but now I know that I have to be careful to avoid sugar for the rest of my life. I don't ever want to experience dumping syndrome again!

I am healed from my surgeries in a physical sense, but this dumping episode proves to me that I will always have to be aware of my weight loss surgery. I can be normal and run with the pack, but I can never forget the extreme measures I have gone through to get to where I am right now.

questions and answers about weight loss surgery

These are the questions that I had and that people ask most frequently on websites.

What are the different kinds of weight loss surgery, and which is the best?

There are primarily three restrictive procedures available in the United States for the surgical control of weight loss: Gastric Bypass (RNY), Vertical Banded Gastroplasty (VBG), and the Laparoscopic Adjustable Gastric Band (Lap-Band).

The Gastric Bypass, Roux-en-Y procedure is considered at this time to be the "gold standard" of bariatric surgery. This procedure reduces the stomach to a small pouch with a capacity to hold only a minimal amount of food, and bypasses a portion of the small intestine to add a mild malabsorptive element, meaning that not even all of the small amount of food eaten can be fully absorbed. Weight loss of 80 to 100 percent of excess body weight is readily achievable for most patients, and long-term maintenance of weight loss has proven to be extremely successful. This procedure provides a very good balance of weight loss, metabolic side effects, and surgical risk.

The Vertical Banded Gastroplasty procedure, also known as gastric stapling, also makes a pouch of the stomach with staples. The drawback to this procedure is that the patient can cheat by eating large amounts of sweets and high calorie liquids, which are processed in the usual manner, often resulting in the patient gaining the weight back. This procedure also has a significant failure rate because of staple line breakdown or band problems.

The Laparoscopic Adjustable Gastric Banding procedure offers another way to limit food intake by placing an adjustable silicon ring completely around the top end of the stomach, creating an hourglass effect. Surgical placement of the band is done laparoscopically and involves no cutting or stapling of the stomach or intestines. The band is inflatable, allowing the surgeon to adjust the size of the band and rate of weight loss by adding or removing fluid from a reservoir just under the skin. Weight loss with the Lap-Band procedure is typically slower and more gradual than with gastric bypass surgery. Since the digestive process remains intact, patients must comply with a strict post-op diet and exercise regimen to achieve and maintain results. The initial U.S. studies, conducted to test the safety of the band for FDA approval, found that most patients lose 26 to 36 percent of their excess weight.

You should discuss all available options with your surgeons and research which procedure is best for your particular medical situation.

What kind of pre-op testing is done?

Most surgeons perform a physical examination along with a blood analysis, urinalysis, arterial blood gas test, electrocardiogram, gall bladder and liver ultrasound, chest X ray, and an upper GI, which is a special set of X rays taken to examine the esophagus, stomach, and small intestine. Of course, more testing may be required if you have additional medical issues such as sleep apnea or a heart condition, and an echocardiogram if you have taken the Fen-Phen combination of weight loss drugs. None of the tests is painful or difficult, but they are time consuming and may take up the better part of a day.

Many surgeons and insurance companies also require a psychological evaluation to determine whether or not you will be able to handle the sometimes difficult lifestyle changes that occur after your surgery. This evaluation is one way of making sure that the individual understands what is required of him or her, and the depth of commitment needed to succeed in both the short- and long-term.

I cannot believe that my mother and sister are giving me such a hard time about my decision to have gastric bypass surgery. How do I deal with the negative comments from friends and family?

I felt very frustrated by my husband's initial comments, "Just eat less," "Why don't you just go on a diet?" and "Why don't you just make believe you had the surgery and eat like you really did?" I came to the conclusion that his comments came from a position of fear and limited understanding of the procedure. The week prior to my surgery, I wrote a heartfelt letter to my father and brother, telling them of my decision to have gastric bypass surgery and why. I explained the possible risks involved and how these risks related to my current co-morbidities. I let them know that I respected any differences of opinion that they might have, and hoped that they would respect my decision. I kept everything very positive, and focused on all the good things that would happen as a result of my having the surgery. I attached links to the before-and-after photo section of the Obesity Help.com website, and profiles of women who were of my approximate size and age. To my surprise, they both responded with great love and support. So my recommendation is to be positive, be strong, be firm, be accepting of others' opinions, but understand that this is a huge decision that only you can make for yourself. In the end, anyone who truly loves you will see the amazing transformation in your health and appearance and be happy for you.

How do I know that my insurance will cover this procedure?

Surgical treatment of morbid obesity is medically necessary because it is the only proven method of achieving long-term weight control. Select a qualified bariatric surgeon and after your consultation, the individual in their office who works directly with the insurance providers will issue a letter of medical necessity to your medical insurance carrier to authorize the procedure. Many times this specialized person in the surgeon's office deals with a specific person at each insurance company and can get an answer in a few days regarding your approval. It generally appears that the larger centers performing more surgeries have better track records in securing insurance authorizations quickly, since they are better tuned into the details of what each insurance carrier requires for approval. There are so many kinds of insurance and so many different versions of each policy that it is difficult to accurately address insurance coverage issues even in general terms.

Now that I have decided to have gastric bypass surgery I can't seem to stop eating. Does everyone look at each meal as a last meal opportunity?

Once I had my date for surgery, every meal was my last meal. I packed on a good 10 to 15 pounds just prior to my surgery, thinking that I would never be able to eat again after my weight loss surgery.

Once you have reached your weight goal there really isn't anything that you can't have at least bite or two of. Just before surgery, I ate huge steaks with fully loaded baked potatoes, piles of fried shrimp, five or six large slices of pizza in a sitting, hunks of cheesecake—and it was all so silly in retrospect. Now that I am at my goal weight, I eat steak, savor a few bites of potato, practically live on shrimp, and occasionally have a small slice of pizza or sugar-free cheesecake, if I choose. I can have a bite or two of anything that I want; my small stomach pouch gives me the control, and I am completely satisfied with just a taste. So my advice is to have a pint of Ben and Jerry's Chubby Hubby, and go to a decadent Sunday brunch buffet at a fancy hotel and get your money's worth for the last time . . . but remember that once you are at your goal weight you can have a little of anything you choose.

What items are important for me to take to the hospital?
I overpacked for my hospital stay and never even opened my small suitcase. Forget the nightgowns, toiletries, and makeup; if you are feeling good enough to care how you look, they will send you home in five minutes. The things that I appreciated and would recommend are:

- Antibacterial wipes: It is very difficult to wash your hands properly with an IV in your forearm or hand. After taking a few laps while pushing your IV pole, touching doorknobs, or being transported via wheelchair for testing, it is good to be able to disinfect your hands.
- Baby wipes: For the first few days it is tough to get around, and it feels good to be able to wash your face and sponge bathe in bed.
- Small squeeze bottle and liquid body soap: If your size causes you to have some difficulty with personal bathroom hygiene, it becomes even more difficult immediately after your surgery and can be very tricky depending on your IV placement. For some, using the moistened baby wipes will be sufficient. You can also fill your squeeze bottle with warm, soapy water and use it to rinse yourself while sitting on the commode. Dry yourself by sitting on a clean towel that you have placed on the side of your hospital bed. In the hospital these squeeze bottles are called "episiotomy bottles" and are commonly used on the maternity floors.

Something comfortable to wear home: You will probably have a drain protruding from your abdomen, and even with a laparoscopic procedure you won't want anything resting on your incisions. You may also be larger than when you checked into the hospital because of bloat and swelling. Pack a pair of sweatpants or leggings with a soft wide waistband to wear rolled below your belly, and a long loose T-shirt that hides everything, along with slip-on shoes.

- Moist and soft lip balm: Your lips will be very crusty and dry after your procedure, and you may not receive a cup of ice chips for some time. Lip balm is priceless in this instance.
- A favorite pillow: It will be difficult to get comfortable in your hospital bed. Having the perfect pillow from your own bed is very reassuring. Press it into your stomach when you have to get out of bed, and hug it to your belly during the car ride home to cushion the impact of road bumps.

What foods should I buy to have in the house when I come home from the hospital?

When you return home from your hospital stay, you just need a few items to sustain you until you are feeling well enough to get out of the house. Remember that you don't eat very much at one time, so you don't need large quantities of the foods you purchase. For the first two to three weeks I ate homemade chicken broth and soups, sugar-free pudding made with skim milk and protein powder, sugar-free ice pops, ricotta cheese, cottage cheese, egg custards, Splenda-sweetened yogurt, the broth from Chinese takeout wonton soup, and homemade applesauce sweetened with Splenda. Toward the end of the third week I added shrimp, salmon, and tuna salads. I also started drinking frosty protein shakes at the end of the second week—they were more appealing than eggs for breakfast.

I was wondering exactly what kind of pain I will experience for the first few days?

When I woke up I wasn't in pain, I just felt incredibly foggy and absolutely terrible. I had nausea and an overall feeling of confusion. I couldn't concentrate on anything anyone said to me, and would fall in and out of consciousness. I wasn't brought back to my room until late in the evening because I was my surgeon's last patient, so the nurses gave me a brief reprieve and allowed me to sleep. My girlfriend Ronni slept in the next bed and I did have to wake her up in the middle of the night so that she could help me use the bathroom. The nurse moved my bed into a sitting position and pulled my legs around so I found myself sitting on the edge of my bed with my feet on the floor. I held a pillow against my abdomen as I stood up. The pain was not debilitating—I rated it a six out of ten. First thing in the morning the nurse helped me out of bed and had me walking around the central nurses' station. I was still very groggy and although I wasn't in much pain, I did have a very hard time staying awake as I walked. My surgeon uses injections and then oral medications for pain management and does not use the morphine pump that some surgeons prefer.

Many of us describe the way we feel the first post-op days in terms of the size of the truck that hit us, but we are talking about an overall dreadful feeling and not one of great pain. This seems to hold true in cases of both laparoscopic and open procedures.

I am four weeks post-op laparoscopic RNY surgery and I have a pain in my left side . . . when will it go away?

The reason your left side hurts is because it is through these openings that most of the laparoscopic action takes place. These are the holes that the larger instruments are manipulated through, so there is more injury to your tissue in this area. It is normal for these sites to cause some discomfort for a few weeks. In order to give them time to heal, it is important that you don't do any lifting or bending while you have this pain; no emptying the dishwasher or the dryer, or picking up the cat dishes from the floor. If you don't already have standing approval from your doctor to take Tylenol, give him a call and follow his recommendation for pain control.

Will I need plastic surgery?

Not everyone desires or even needs reconstructive plastic surgery after the large weight loss following gastric bypass surgery. Factors such as age, your starting weight, and where you carried the bulk of your excess weight all influence the potential for your skin to recoil to normal tone once you near your ideal weight. In the average patient, there is often an excess of body skin and fatty tissue. In the area of the belly and back, this excess of abdominal apron skin may be appropriately treated using procedures such as an *abdominoplasty* or *panniculectomy*. In more extreme excess skin situations, especially where the excess is circular in nature involving the belly, hips, back, buttocks, and outer thighs, a more extensive procedure is available. This procedure is called a *belt lipectomy* and is like a face-lift for the torso. Both males and females may have excessive hanging breast tissue that can be reconstructed during a *breast lift* procedure. Some patients will have hanging tissue of the upper arms called "bat wings," which can be removed during a procedure called *brachioplasty*. Some patients will choose to undergo a *thigh lift* for the removal of the hanging folds of skin on their inner and outer thighs. Brachioplasty and thigh lift procedures are not usually "favorite" procedures of plastic surgeons, as there are no natural folds in these areas in which to hide the long scars, so make sure your surgeon is practiced in these particular procedures.

In any case, make sure that you choose your plastic or reconstructive surgeon as wisely as you chose your weight loss surgeon. Make sure that your plastic surgeon is recognized by the American Board of

Plastic Surgery as board certified. It is also important that you know that your plastic surgeon has regularly performed the procedure you are considering, and it is one of her specialties. It is helpful if the plastic surgeon is familiar with the specific challenges that weight loss surgery patients present, as our considerable amount of excess skin can be more difficult to reconstruct.

As I approached my goal weight, even regular exercise had not reduced the apron of skin hanging from my abdomen. Although this excess skin didn't medically compromise my life, I was unhappy with the way it looked. My surgeon performed an extended abdominoplasty panniculectomy, in which the lower abdominal incision runs about six inches past each of my hipbones, and allowed my surgeon to excise excess skin from my flanks in addition to my front belly area. This is the most common reconstructive procedure performed after weight loss surgery. My abdominal reconstruction was considered cosmetic and was not a covered benefit of my insurance.

If you are considering reconstructive surgery once you have lost your weight, make sure that you visit your dermatologist if you suffer from any infections or rashes in your folds of skin, so that these problems can be noted on your medical chart. This may help you to prove to your insurance company that skin removal is medically necessary in your case.

Does it hurt to have the staples removed?
Not only did it not hurt to have the staples removed, it didn't even pinch or feel funny. It was much better than I anticipated. The dot marks from the staples were the only scars that I had left. After only two weeks, my incisions had almost disappeared. If I look at my almost three-year post-op belly, I honestly can only locate one laparoscopic incision.

I am ten days post-op and cry when I see Burger King commercials on TV. What have I done to myself?

You haven't healed enough to be able to eat anything even resembling food, you are totally exhausted from your surgery, and your emotions are out of control—so it is not out of the question that you would sit around thinking how much you miss your old best friend, food. At this point you haven't lost a measurable amount of weight *and* you can't eat, so you have nothing. Once you have lost 65 or so pounds, you won't care as much about food, and by then you will be able to eat a little and won't think about what you are missing. Hang in there; I promise that it gets much, much better. I understand that it is terrible right now, but that will soon change and you will be able to laugh about the thought of crying over pictures of a Whopper! Soon you will reach that defining moment where the scale tips just enough in your favor for you to understand the meaning of "Nothing tastes as good as thin feels," and then it really gets exciting.

I am only a week post-op and I can drink an entire protein shake. Have I stretched out my pouch?

You cannot stretch out your pouch with liquids. It is simply impossible. It pours in and dribbles out. If you are sipping slowly, it is smoothly running in and out of your pouch. Even if the drain in the sink is half closed, the liquid won't back up as long as you are pouring it in gradually. Once you start eating more solid foods, like shrimp or chicken, you will see just how small your pouch is and that it is intact.

I am two months post-op and I have only lost 38 pounds. I am nervous and upset most of the time, as I am afraid that I will be the only one that this surgery doesn't work for. Does anyone else have these feelings?

Calm down and take a deep breath. You are just getting to the point where you have recovered from major surgery. As far as your weight loss, losing 38 pounds in two months is fantastic. We all have those moments when we think that we are the only one who isn't going to lose weight—that is normal considering our pitiful track records of losing weight and keeping it off. Some of us are faster losers from the start; others are slow and steady. Most of us even out over the course of that first year to similar totals. Don't put any added stress on yourself. Just remember to keep away from the carbs, start being aware of getting in more protein each day, start moving toward drinking eight cups of water a day, move around a little, and you will get there.

I think that it would really help you to join an on-line support group like the one at ObesityHelp.com and keep a journal of your feelings and progress. You would be amazed at how many people feel exactly the way that you do at this very minute. When I had just returned home from the hospital, it made me feel connected to see all the others who were at the same stage and were living through identical situations. I had started keeping an on-line journal on the website before my surgery, and when I didn't post for a few days, people who were following my progress sent me e-mails asking how I was doing. I had friends that I didn't even know about! I talked via posts with women who were a few steps ahead of me, and they were eager to give me the heads-up for what to expect. I had people to talk to who were at various steps on the same journey. The photo galleries were an amazing source of strength for me. If I had the tiniest seed of self-doubt all I had to do was click on a few of the members' before-and-after pictures and I would have tears of happiness streaming down my face in minutes. Those pictures would give me enough fuel to get through anything in my path. Give it a try and you will see that going through this solo is not the way to do it.

In three months I have lost 41 pounds, but it isn't as much as I had hoped to lose; do you have any suggestions for keeping motivated?

Congratulations on losing 41 pounds, you are doing great. There is not a time limit or set schedule for pounds lost. We tend to put negative pressure on ourselves because we are so used to being failures at dieting. Don't set unrealistic expectations for weight loss and don't be too tough on yourself. Keep your focus on the long term and remember that these 41 pounds are gone forever this time.

To keep motivated, make sure that you attend your surgeon's monthly support group meetings; these groups are essential lifelines for bariatric surgery patients. If your surgeon does not have a live support group set up, then make sure that you join an on-line weight loss support system such as the message board at ObesityHelp.com or SpotlightHealth.com. These groups give you an outlet to share your feelings and deepest fears, they let you know that you are not alone, and they connect you to others in the exact same situation.

I am five months post-op and when I was washing my hair this morning, my fingers were completely tangled with hair that had fallen out. Help, my hair is falling out, what should I do?

I also lost what seemed to be a lot of hair during my fifth post-op month. It started out slowly and increased until I was in panic mode, running out and buying Biotin and adding a second 50-gram protein shake to my diet. I have a very knowledgeable dermatologist and he assured me that almost everyone who has a major operation would notice increased hair shedding for a few months afterward. On top of the shock of the surgery, our food intake plummets and we essentially develop protein malnutrition. The body then attempts to reserve protein by shifting the growing hairs into a resting phase. Massive hair shedding can occur two to three months later and even the remaining hair can be pulled out by the roots fairly easily. Once we rebound and begin to eat more protein, the condition reverses itself. For those of you who are considering this surgery, it is alarming seeing the hair in your drain. But as part of the big picture, it isn't that big a deal and doesn't happen to everyone. By the end of my seventh post-op month, I had a head full of one-inch sprouts peeking through my longer hair! I am not trying to discount the impact of this hair loss, but it is temporary and does start to grow back very quickly. Fortunately it occurred at the time when I had lost enough weight and didn't focus as much on the hair loss. Friends weren't looking at my hair—they were noticing my incredible shrinking body. I took the opportunity to have a makeover and had my hairdresser give me a new, stylish, shorter look that I would never have tried at 278 pounds. My dermatologist insists that specialty shampoos and special vitamin preparations have no impact on the process, and are a waste of money.

I'm almost one year out . . . when does your self-image change? I am happy to be 165 pounds instead of 310, but I still see nothing but fat when I look in the mirror.
This is a common feeling that echoes in our monthly support group meetings. I'm sure it has a lot to do with a lifetime of seeing ourselves in a negative light and as quickly as we all lose weight, our minds just don't have enough time to adjust to the physical change. We still see ourselves as fat because we are still the same person on the inside, looking at the world through the same eyes and anticipating certain behaviors from others. Now that we are wearing size 10 clothes, we realize that we aren't supermodels, we are real women and men, with curves, lumps, and wrinkles, and we are disappointed instead of being

proud of our amazing success. I compare myself to photos of my girl-friends rather than the girls in the magazines to better center myself. This weight comes off so fast that we expect miracles, and if our life isn't suddenly transformed, we start to feel as if we are failures. Keep focusing on the great things that are happening for you, affirm your successes, celebrate every new step you have the courage to take, and you will find that it is so easy to love yourself.

Do I have to take multivitamins, iron, B-12, and calcium forever?

According to bariatric experts, the condition of morbid obesity is usually already accompanied by dietary vitamin and mineral deficiencies. Following surgery, gastric bypass patients typically experience additional nutritional deficiencies as this procedure induces a state of semi-starvation; we simply cannot ingest enough food to give our bodies sufficient nutrients. The typical gastric bypass procedure takes off-line the portion of the intestine responsible for the absorption of vitamin A, vitamin B-12, calcium, iron and, because the intrinsic factor-producing area of the stomach is bypassed by food, B-12 deficiencies are common. The gastric bypass procedure reduces fat absorption, and along with it the absorption of fat-soluble vitamins including beta-carotene, vitamin D, vitamin E, and vitamin K. Protein deficiencies, the inability to tolerate red meats, and reduced use of dairy products combined with a drastic reduction in the amounts of fruits and vegetables eaten, may be responsible for low blood and tissue levels of calcium, iron, magnesium, potassium, and zinc. The limited use of dairy products and/or lactose intolerance further reduces the calcium position of the bariatric patient. The lack of digestive enzymes and stomach acids coming into contact with food also play an important role in mineral absorption.

After surgery, it is important for us to follow up with our surgical team in order to remain healthy. Our lab values must be monitored to make sure our blood levels are sufficient and, if not, supplemented to keep problems from occurring. Lifelong supplements of multivitamins, iron if needed, B-12, and calcium are mandatory following gastric bypass surgery.

After my surgery I took Flintstones Complete chewable vitamins because they gave me the assurance that nothing would get stuck in my new pouch opening. I thought that they provided basic nutrients in the most absorbable form. For the first year I had too much to think about with making good food choices and eating enough protein to consider the fact that just as I don't metabolize all of the food I eat, that this would apply to the children's vitamins I was taking. I didn't like eating a handful of Tums every day as a calcium supplement, so many days I didn't bother, but I did occasionally pop a B-12 tablet under my tongue. It wasn't until proper eating became less of an effort that the importance of taking my supplements and carefully monitoring my blood levels registered with me.

I have noticed that several of my weight loss surgery contemporaries have deficiencies, most notably anemia. This has made me rethink the whole supplement issue and how our choices can affect our long-term health. I now realize not only how important it is to take supplements but also the ones that are specifically designed for our altered digestive systems. It's not which vitamins we take—it's how much our bodies absorb. I wish I had this epiphany when I was newly post-op. I chose to have this surgery to be healthy and fit, yet for almost 24 months I took vitamins designed for a 40-pound child.

The line of supplements produced by VistaVitamins has been specifically formulated to meet the unique nutritional requirements and address the absorption challenges of gastric bypass patients. Vista-Vitamins uses the highest quality ingredients, specifically chosen to improve absorbability, and patented mineral amino acid chelates from Albion Laboratories.

Protein is made up of chains of amino acids. The body is very efficient at absorbing amino acids during the process of digestion.

When the tiny, organic mineral molecules become surrounded by and bonded to an amino acid, this is called chelation. This amino acid shell allows the mineral to be smuggled across the intestinal lining and into the system. VistaVitamins uses these principles to gain maximum absorption and efficiency from the minerals in their supplements.

The best feature of VistaVitamins supplements is that everything we need is contained in one formula; there is no need to purchase multiple bottles of vitamins, minerals, sublingual B-12 tablets, Tums, or giant calcium citrate pills. Since I started taking VistaVitamins, I haven't missed a dose and the increased absorption is obvious to me in the renewed thickness of my hair, strength of my nails, and increased energy. I take the Wellness Plus capsules, but there is also a Chewable Wellness tablet that has slight variations in its formula for early post-op patients. This is an excellent and important product for anyone having gastric bypass surgery.

What kind of calcium is the best one for us to take, calcium carbonate or calcium citrate?

There is a great deal of debate regarding this important topic since the wrong choice of supplements may manifest itself as severe osteoporosis years from now when it is too late to reverse its effects. Why the debate? Many surgeons simply recommend that their gastric bypass patients take Tums, which are calcium carbonate. Calcium carbonate is inexpensive and is used in many of the calcium-enriched foods in grocery stores, so it is readily available. While calcium carbonate is adequate for most people to use to supplement their diet, calcium citrate is a better form of calcium for gastric bypass patients, as we no longer have the necessary stomach acids in our pouches or bypassed intestines that facilitate calcium carbonate absorption.

The National Institutes of Health, in its Consensus Statement regarding Optimal Calcium Uptake clearly makes the case for calcium citrate.

Absorption of one form of calcium supplementation, calcium carbonate, is impaired in fasted individuals who have an absence of gastric acid. Alternatively, calcium supplementation in the form of calcium citrate does not require gastric acid for optimal absorption and thus could be considered in individuals with reduced gastric acid production.

Additionally, the University of Pittsburgh Medical Center has recently published the results of a study "Bone Loss Associated with Weight Loss After Stomach Reduction Surgery." Dr. Penelope Coates, M.D., postdoctoral fellow at the University of Pittsburgh Medical Center's Osteoporosis Prevention and Treatment Center, has discovered that women and men who have stomach reduction surgery to lose weight may be losing bone mass even when they take daily calcium supplements, putting them at risk for osteoporosis and bone fracture.

We have been recommending that people take 1000 mg calcium citrate daily because we were concerned that calcium carbonate would not be absorbed after the surgery. The calcium in Tums is calcium carbonate. Our patients were taking a variety of supplements but have largely switched to calcium citrate.

With the growing popularity of VistaVitamins Wellness Formula supplements, which are made specifically for the gastric bypass surgery patient, there is another form of calcium that is worth taking note of. Studies have shown that Albion Laboratories patented calcium amino acid chelate, Chelazome, is absorbed approximately 1.83 times er than calcium citrate and its bioavailability is even higher than the calcium in milk. I use VistaVitamins Wellness Plus Formula, which contains this highly absorbable form of calcium in the easy-to-swallow capsules that I take twice daily, making a separate calcium supplement unnecessary.

If you are following your surgeon's program of vitamin supplementation and need a good separate calcium citrate supplement, I recommend the liquid suspension from Tropical Oasis. One tablespoon gives you 1200 mg of calcium citrate daily. Before switching to VistaVitamins, I kept a bottle of Tropical Oasis Calcium Magnesium Citrate in my refrigerator; the fresh tart orange yogurt taste is actually delicious. Since it is recommended that we take our calcium in small increments, take one-half tablespoon each morning and one-half tablespoon before bed.

How can I swallow my pills when I can't drink enough water to get them down?

Immediately post-op I would bury my pills in a spoonful of sugar-free Jell-O instant pudding. I kept a bowl in the refrigerator just for taking pills. Something about the smooth, thick texture made it easier for me than water, since I could only take baby sips of water. The small pills I could take whole; larger ones I would cut into quarters.

Why drink so much water?

When you are losing weight, there is a heavy load of waste products to eliminate, mostly in the urine. Some of these substances can form crystals, which can cause kidney stones. Drinking lots of water helps your body to efficiently rid itself of waste products, promoting better weight loss. Water will also fill your stomach, and will help to prolong your sense of satisfaction with food. If you are hungry and have the desire to eat between meals, drinking cold water will help you to control the hunger. Most nutritional specialists agree that gastric bypass patients need at least eight cups of water each day.

What's so important about exercise?

When you have a gastric bypass, you lose weight because the amount of food energy that you eat is much less than what your body needs to operate. It has to make up the difference by burning reserves. If you do not exercise daily, your body will metabolize your unused muscle, and you will lose muscle mass and strength. Daily aerobic exercise for at least twenty minutes will communicate to your body that you want to use your muscles, and force it to burn the fat instead. The idea of having this operation is to become slender and healthy, not scrawny and weak. If you lose most of your excess fat, and retain most of your muscles, imagine how much power and energy you will have to enjoy your reclaimed life.

What are some good low-carb protein foods I can grab for a quick breakfast or lunch?

It is easy to find healthy foods that are easy to prepare and eat on the run if you have given it some advance thought. Possibilities include cottage cheese, ricotta cheese, string cheese, a rolled-up piece of deli turkey or ham, tuna salad on a melba thin, cooked and peeled shrimp, beef jerky, a few nuts, a deviled egg, a cube of feta cheese, a few roasted soy nuts, thinly sliced leftover steak, thinly sliced grilled Italian sausage, an egg custard. For breakfast, blend some ricotta or cottage cheese with a little Smucker's Light Sugar Free Apricot Preserves and pile it on half of a Wasa cinnamon flat bread. For a great light lunch, scoop some ricotta cheese into a small dish, add a little Newman's Own spaghetti sauce, sprinkle with some chopped string cheese and Parmesan, then microwave until bubbly.

When can I have a few vegetables? I am craving some salad.

Once you have gotten through the initial few weeks of intense healing and have started to get comfortable with eating again, it is all right to add in a few bites of very low carbohydrate vegetables after you eat your needed protein. Once I was two months post-op and was doing well in eating my small portions of shrimp salad and softly cooked salmon, I added a small handful of lightly dressed baby salad greens to my plate and would chew a tender leaf with a few of my bites of food. I would cook a few baby spinach leaves with my shrimp in a little garlic and olive oil; the spinach shreds would add moisture to the mouthful and make it even easier to eat. Just make sure that you choose low-carb vegetables, and that you eat four or five bites of protein for every one bite of vegetable. A tablespoon of sautéed, seasoned spinach or a few bites of baby lettuce leaves add less than one gram of carbohydrate to your daily tally, so even surgeons with the strictest nutritional regimen would agree with this one.

Can I drink soda after surgery?

Once you are comfortable with eating regular foods, are doing well with drinking eight glasses of water a day, and have become accustomed to your new digestive system, having a diet soda now and then will not harm you, or your operation. Some doctors tell their patients to avoid diet soda because it is easy to fall back into those old bad habits of drinking multiple cans of soda. Tastes and sensations change so much after surgery that some things that we loved pre-op are very unappealing afterward. The carbonation in diet soda produces a tremendous amount of gas in our pouch, which is extremely unpleasant. I tried a sip of diet cola when I was about five months post-op because we were on the road and the gas station didn't have cold bottles of water. The first sip foamed up in my stomach and I felt like it was coming out of my mouth. It was so dreadful that I wasn't interested in another sip. Now that I am more than two years post-op, I occasionally enjoy a diet soda, but I will pour it from a height of about twelve inches into an oversized glass filled with ice to flatten out most of the carbonation.

Ever since my surgery I have a gurgling sound when I swallow and terrible burping when I eat or drink. Is something wrong?

The gurgles or burps in your esophagus and stomach are normal. You used to have a big stomach bag for all that air and food to roll around in. Now that your stomach is a tiny pouch, there just isn't much space for the air you were unaware that you were gulping. Just be more conscious of taking in extra air while you are eating and drinking and it will lessen.

Once in a while a food will make me sick but when I throw it up, there is so much spit and mucus. Does this happen to everyone?

When we eat something that our stomach cannot handle, the problem gets compounded when the undigested food is quickly dumped into our intestines. The intestines draw water from the bloodstream in an attempt to dilute the offending food. This creates the excessive mucus and slime. I find that this happens if I eat too fast, don't chew well, or continue to eat when I am already full, so it definitely serves as negative reinforcement for me!

How do you make good choices when you are not eating at home?

In order to make good food choices, you have to give it a little thought and use your imagination. If your grandmother makes lasagna, just eat the ground meat and cheese. If they serve Italian subs at your co-worker's baby shower, roll up a couple of pieces of cold meat and enjoy it. If your Dad makes his famous fried fish, break it in half, eat the tender, moist pieces from the center, and leave the breading. If your friends vote to have Chinese food before the movie, drink the broth from the hot-and-sour soup, eat the shrimp, a couple of pieces of tender vegetables, and leave the rice. If you are at a steakhouse, order the scallop appetizer or shrimp cocktail as your dinner, and if you are at least seven to eight months post-op have a few thin slices of someone's tender filet. If you are traveling and get locked into a situation where there just isn't anything healthy for you to eat, break out your stash of protein bars. I can't tell you how many times I nibbled a coconut protein bar while everyone else was chowing down on greasy chicken wings and deep-fried mozzarella sticks.

Do I really need to go to the support group meetings?

The support group meetings are a very important part of our physical and emotional healing process. Even though I was able to easily adjust to post-op life, there were still times when I noticed a particular pain or hiccup, or had terrible feelings of self-doubt after experiencing a temporary stall in weight loss. Being able to share my thoughts and experiences with a roomful of people who understood what I was going through made the journey easier. I also felt that it helped me to share my discoveries and celebrate my successes with my peers. The surgeons operated on our bodies, not our brains, and I really look forward to the positive reinforcement of my monthly meeting with my new weight-loss friends.

What did you do with your old clothes?

Like many serial yo-yo dieters, I had a closet full of clothes in various sizes and styles. One of the first things I tackled when I started to feel better was to organize my closet by size. I was amazed at how fast I was dropping sizes. Once I was safely out of a size, I would list each item on the clothing exchange on the ObesityHelp.com website. There were so many women who were happily melting into my size 28s or 20s after starting their journey at even higher weights. I developed a rapport with several ladies who liked the designer names that I wore, and I would box up my entire season of a particular size of business and casual wear and send it to them. They in turn would advertise the clothing on the exchange when they had melted out of that size and ship it off to someone else. It is a great way to empty your closets, as you'll quickly find out that none of your still-heavy friends will want your clothes once you are smaller than they are.

What was the thing that surprised you the most in the first year of your weight loss?

My husband's daughter Dione had mailed me a pair of size 8 Calvin Klein Capri jeans and a disposable camera in a package that were waiting for me when I came home from the hospital. I started to cry when I saw the tiny little pants and held them up to my huge body. I looked at my husband and just shook my head and laughed to hide the pain in knowing that I would never fit into those pants. There was a letter in the package, instructing me to have Ty take a photo of me right now and then on each month's anniversary date for the next year, so that I would never forget what I went through. There was no way that I wanted to have my picture taken in my huge flowered robe with my bloated belly, but my husband kept on it and I finally gave in. Every month on the 11th, there he was with that camera to take my picture. After taking the last picture, I dropped off the camera but didn't pick up the photos for several months.

I actually have two things that surprised me during the first year of my weight loss. The first is that I actually lost enough weight to slip into those size 8 pants. I will be particularly humble while I'm wearing them this summer.

The second is that it is incredible to have a photo journal of my progress during those months of losing such a large amount of weight. It was so thoughtful, and it was not something that I would have ever done on my own. It took me a while to get up the courage to pick up the pictures—the reality of what I looked like was truly shocking—but I am so proud of all that I went through to get where I am right now.

protein, carbohydrates, and sugar after weight loss surgery

Protein

Protein is critical for repairing and replacing cell tissue as well as building new muscle. When we have major surgery such as the RNY gastric bypass procedure, protein is necessary so tissues can heal. Immediately after RNY surgery, it is nearly impossible for us to ingest adequate protein through foods alone, which is why many surgeons recommend that patients consume protein supplements via shakes. It is good nutrition for us to be able to rely on a daily protein supplement of 25 to 50 grams and add to it with high-protein, low-fat, and lower carbohydrate foods.

How do you determine the right amount of protein for yourself? An active person needs around 1.25 grams of protein per kilogram of ideal body weight (1 kilogram equals 2.2 pounds, so divide your goal weight by 2.2). We use a person's ideal body weight to calculate protein targets because fat tissue does not need protein. Therefore a person currently weighing 247 pounds who exercises and has an ideal body weight of 145 would need 82 grams of protein daily to maintain their muscle mass and good health (145 pounds divided by 2.2 pounds per kilograms then multiplied by 1.25 grams per kilogram). A person currently weighing 341 pounds with an ideal body weight of 185 would need 105 grams of protein daily to maintain muscle mass and good health (185 pounds divided by 2.2 pounds per kilogram then multiplied by 1.25 grams per kilogram).

Note that these figures are the recommended grams of protein needed for good nutrition and to keep our muscles intact. We want to

...le. Our vital organs are made of muscle, and need ...n efficiently. So when we talk about 65 to 100 grams ...his is not a high protein diet, it is minimum fulfillment ...ein needs. Too little protein is a serious concern as it ...s the incidence of osteoporosis, which is why appropriate calcium supplements are also an important part of our diet.

Not only does adequate protein fend off muscle loss, but it can also speed up our fat-burning processes. Protein has the highest thermal effect of any food. This means that protein foods speed up your metabolism because your body has to work harder to digest, process, and use this nutrient compared to fat or carbohydrate. Use solid protein such as fish or meats as the main part of each of your three daily meals. Proteins take longer to digest and they are absorbed more slowly by your body, giving you a longer-lasting, steady source of energy.

Just as important to losing weight is the very important inhibitory effect protein has on the craving for more food. Protein is more filling and therefore we are satisfied more quickly and for a longer period with a protein meal than we would be with a high-carbohydrate meal.

Be proactive, be accountable for your health, and make sure you are getting enough protein! Grab a protein bar or a slice of turkey breast instead of a cracker or high-carb snack. Eat the protein on your plate before you even think of touching the carbohydrate.

Protein Foods Serving size	grams of protein	grams of carbohydrate
½ cup low fat yogurt	6.5	8
½ cup 2 percent milk	4.0	6
½ cup 2 percent cottage cheese	16.0	5
½ cup part skim ricotta	14.0	6
1 ounce provolone cheese	7.0	.5
1 ounce mozzarella cheese	8.0	.8
2 ounces sliced deli ham	14.5	0
2 ounces sliced deli turkey	13.0	0

Serving size	grams of protein	grams of carbohydrate
3 ounces lean ground beef, grilled	22.0	0
3 ounces beef sirloin, grilled	26.0	0
3 ounces roasted chicken, dark	22.0	0
3 ounces roasted chicken, white	26.0	0
3 ounces roasted turkey, dark	24.0	0
3 ounces roasted turkey, white	25.0	0
½ cup chicken salad	18.0	1
3 ounces broiled sole	21.0	0
3 ounces grilled tuna	23.0	0
3 ounces broiled halibut	23.0	0
3 ounces broiled red snapper	22.0	0
3 ounces broiled scallops, sautéed	18.0	2
3 ounces shrimp, peeled, steamed	21.0	1
3 ounces water-pack tuna	22.0	0
1 large egg	7.0	.5
¼ cup almonds	7.0	7
2 tablespoons peanut butter	8.5	6

Carbohydrates

Carbohydrates are easily and readily absorbed by the body for immediate energy. When you eat a carbohydrate-loaded food, it is quickly metabolized, driving up blood sugar levels. Your body immediately responds by releasing insulin to send your blood sugar back down. This is why a slab of warm bread, muffins, or a high-sugar food gives you a quick energy burst that soon gives way to a sluggish and tired feeling. This cycle of blood sugar highs and lows creates highs and lows of hunger. Even though you have just eaten a carbohydrate snack of crackers and are full, you are quickly hungry again because there is little lasting satisfaction in this quick fix. In addition, instead of drawing on stored fat reserves for your energy, your body burned the food you just consumed.

When you burn more calories than you consume, your body must draw on reserves to keep you going. According to acknowledged medical principles, when you cut back your intake of carbohydrates, your body converts from the metabolic process of burning carbohydrate to burning your stored fat as its primary energy source. The stored fat easily metabolizes into the components that supply energy for the body's cells, resulting in weight loss. Many of the top bariatric surgeons recommend that those of us who have RNY gastric bypass surgery consume less than 25 grams of carbohydrate per day to push our body to burn this warehoused fat for energy.

In the first few days at home after our RNY surgery, it is acceptable to have a few of the higher carbohydrate foods as our first foods, so that we get used to eating again. A little potato soup, or a few bites of bean puree or hummus are higher in carbohydrates, but are safe, soft foods that will not burden our swollen stomach and intestines. We really cannot ingest enough of these higher carbohydrate foods at this point to hurt us. By the time we start to feel better, we become aware of protein and can redirect our diets.

Our surgeons and nutritionists all tell us to eat protein first, but as we heal and get back into cooking for our families, preparing meals for ourselves, and eating in restaurants, we need to know how to choose foods that will keep carbohydrate consumption to a minimum. Generally speaking, any food that comes from a growing plant or is processed from a product grown in the ground is a carbohydrate. Milk and dairy products are also included because they contain lactose ("milk sugar"). We are looking for the highest protein, vitamins, and minerals for the lowest amount of carbs. Fortunately, some of the most nutritious vegetables and fruits have the lowest carbohydrate counts. I have included a basic list of lower-carb vegetables. Usually the more watery or acidic vegetables are lower, while the starchier or sweeter vegetables are higher in carbs. If you can choose either a small dish of zucchini or half of a baked potato, the zucchini is a much better choice as it provides fiber, vitamins, and other nutrients, but very few carbohydrates. The potato provides too few nutrients to warrant using up your entire daily carbohydrate budget. A ¼-cup portion of spinach sautéed with garlic is packed with nutrients, whereas an equal amount of pasta salad provides nothing of consequence but unwanted carbohydrates. A few cubes of tomato tossed with shredded romaine are a much better choice than a small dish of corn in terms of nutrition. Sautéed sliced asparagus have fiber and a high nutritional value when compared to a scoop of rice or a small dinner roll. Look at your 25 grams of daily carbohydrates as an allowance and make good choices to spend your carbohydrate grams wisely, choosing vegetables and fruits that provide the most nutrients in combination with the fewest grams of carbohydrate. Eating after RNY gastric bypass surgery is all about making good choices. Have a bite of the baked potato or pasta salad if you need to satisfy your taste for it, but be aware of the tradeoff you are making and have a few bites of the more nutritious selection as well.

Vegetable Carbohydrate Counts

		grams of carbohydrate
Arugula	½ cup baby leaves, raw	0.4
Romaine	½ cup shredded, raw	0.6
Mushrooms	¼ cup sliced, raw	0.7
Bok Choy	¼ cup sliced, cooked	0.7
Cucumber	¼ cup sliced, raw	0.7
Cabbage	¼ cup shredded, raw	0.8
Radishes	¼ cup sliced, raw	1.0
Asparagus	2 medium spears, cooked	1.2
Zucchini	¼ cup sliced, cooked	1.3
Cauliflower	¼ cup chopped, cooked	1.5
Spinach	¼ cup chopped, cooked	1.6
Fennel	¼ cup sliced, cooked	1.6
Eggplant	¼ cup diced, cooked	1.6
Swiss Chard	¼ cup sliced, cooked	1.8

		grams of carbohydrate
Tomato	¼ cup diced, raw or canned	1.8
Broccoli	¼ cup chopped, cooked	1.9
Green Beans	¼ cup sliced, cooked	2.3
Collard Greens	¼ cup chopped, cooked	2.3
Green Pepper	¼ cup diced, raw	2.4
Avocado	¼ small Hass variety	3.2
Onion	¼ cup chopped, raw	3.2
Artichoke Hearts	¼ cup sliced, canned	4.1
Carrots	¼ cup sliced, cooked	4.1
Peas	¼ cup cooked	5.0
Brussels Sprouts	4 small whole	7.8
Corn	¼ cup kernels, cooked	10.6
Sweet Potato	½ small, roasted	13.9
Potato	½ small, baked	25.4

Fruit Carbohydrate Counts

		grams of carbohydrate
Strawberries	½ cup sliced, fresh	2.9
Raspberries	½ cup whole, fresh	3.5
Plum	½ small 2-inch fruit	4.2
Peach	½ small 2½-inch fruit	4.3
Watermelon	½ cup small cubes	5.1
Blueberries	¼ cup whole, fresh	5.1
Orange	¼ cup chopped sections	5.3
Kiwi	½ whole fruit	5.6
Cherries	¼ cup pitted, fresh	6.0
Cantaloupe	½ cup small cubes	6.6
Honeydew	½ cup small cubes	7.8
Nectarine	½ small 2½-inch fruit	8.0

Apple	½ small 2½ -inch fruit	9.5
Pineapple	½ cup cubes, fresh/canned in juice	9.6
Pear, fresh	½ small	10.7
Pear, canned	½ cup, diced, no sugar added	14.2
Banana	½ cup, sliced	15.8
Grapes	½ cup seedless, white or red	15.8
Banana	1 small 6–7 inch, whole	23.0

Sugar and Dumping Syndrome

If people who have had RNY gastric bypass surgery eat foods with high levels of sugar or fat, we risk experiencing the wrath of "dumping syndrome." When we ingest a high volume of sugar or fat our body attempts to dilute the food by drawing large amounts of liquid into the intestine from the blood. This causes a rapid drop in blood pressure and a significant rise in blood sugar, which in turn prods the pancreas to release insulin. This insulin release is so strong that it sends the now-high blood sugar levels plummeting, causing a combination of intense nausea, profuse sweating, faintness, weakness, severe and immediate intestinal cramping, and then explosive diarrhea. Most people who have experienced it say it is so awful that they will do any-thing they can to avoid it again. I experienced a mild dumping episode only once and it is one of the most unpleasant physical experiences I have ever had.

People who have had RNY gastric bypass surgery must always monitor their sugar intake. Be proactive and become a relentless label reader, since sugar is found in products that you would never suspect. There are excellent sugar-free products to satisfy an occasional desire for something sweet, so we don't need to sabotage our success by pushing the envelope and discovering our dumping level. I would rather not know exactly how much sugar triggers my mechanism; the fear of dumping keeps me from eating a hunk of layer cake. Dumping provides strong negative feedback and therefore limits the undesirable behavior. A weight-loss surgery friend of mine who is now at her goal weight says, "Dumping is like having a personal food cop with you at all times so you can't hide in your closet and eat like you did pre-op." Limit your sugar intake to less than 5 to 8 grams at one time, at the end of a meal, to err on the side of caution. It is believed that dumping occurs when the sugar load is greater than 15 grams at one time, but tolerance levels can and will vary. Dumping can also occur when we eat too much of any food, but it is most common with sugar and fat.

If we make good choices a part of our lives now, it will make us long-term success stories in weight-loss surgery history. If we make bad choices now while we are severely limited in our stomach capacity, what choices will we make when we can eat larger portions in two years? If you are regularly eating 125 grams of carbohydrate in a day and have discovered that you do not "dump" on sugar at three months post-op, what will you be eating at eighteen months post-op? If we change our relationship with food now, it will be second nature to us in the future, and we will never have to diet again.

protein shakes

For the first weeks after surgery, the stomach pouch and the *stoma*, or opening, into the intestine are very swollen and small. I started drinking protein shakes within days of returning home from the hospital and have had one a day ever since. The cold frostiness was soothing to my stomach and it took the place of my morning coffee while I read my e-mail. There are so many people who have had their surgery, try one shake, decide they don't like the taste or texture, and that is it for the protein supplements. You owe it to yourself and your dedication to your health to figure out a way to make these shakes a part of your life. People who hated protein shakes love them once they follow my suggestions and recipes to the letter.

I have tried many different varieties of protein powder, and I have found that I prefer Zero Carb Isopure when I am making a frosty, thick blender shake. The pure whey isolate used by Isopure is not at all gritty or chalky, the smooth powder dissolves completely, and there is no aftertaste. Two scoops provide 50 grams of protein, and an excellent source of vitamins and minerals. Vanilla allows you to layer on flavor and go in many directions, whereas a three-pound canister of chocolate or strawberry is more limiting.

With the recent focus on obesity, the health food and protein shake market is expanding so rapidly that it is easy to get confused. Every time I go to the nutrition store there are new and better products on the shelves. I stand in the aisle poring over labels like I am in a bookstore. I buy every new low-carb, no-sugar protein powder and bar, then experiment with different shake flavors. I knew early on that for my own health I would need to develop a long-term love of protein shakes and keep in touch with the most up-to-date products on the market. This is the reason I have developed a website, www.Bariatric Eating.com, so that surgical post-ops will have a place to find the best current protein products for our specific dietary needs (see Sources, page 246). No matter which brand you decide tastes best, make sure your protein powder is a no- or very low-carbohydrate powder; there are formulations made for weight gain and bodybuilding that are high-carbohydrate mixtures containing sugar that are not good for gastric bypass patients. There are hidden carbohydrates, fat, and sugar in products you would never think of, so again, become a dedicated label reader.

I think a Zero Carb Isopure Creamy Vanilla shake tastes pretty good as is, but a few low-carb ingredients can turn a plain vanilla shake into a concoction that tastes like it came from Dairy Queen. Too much fruit, however, could make you dump, and adding too many extras can turn a healthy drink into a very high-carbohydrate, high-calorie smoothie, so don't go crazy.

Texture is important when making a great-tasting protein shake. If you turn on the blender and leave it on high, the shake will get very dense and foamy, giving you a huge volume full of air, that is almost unpleasant to drink. If you pulse the blender on and off, the shake will have less volume and a frosty, milkshake consistency.

There are two new lines of proteins that blend well simply using a small covered shaker and some ice. ProPlete Gold is an excellent product that quickly and easily blends into a delicious shake. The fruit flavors have small pieces of dried fruit mixed in and the chocolate is dark and rich. I highly recommend this very good tasting protein powder if you find that a thin shake is more appealing to your changing tastes. Nectar is also a hot product on the low-carb protein scene as it is one of the first whey proteins that mixes into a sweet yet puckery Kool-Aid-type fruit drink. I mix it with water and crushed ice in my sports bottle and drink it on the way to the gym or to the beach. It is very refreshing (see Sources, page 246).

Resist the urge to add lots of milk when making a shake, or you will have to deal with drinking a quart of protein shake. A low volume of liquid results in a smaller glass of shake with the same protein and nutrients. Also, be aware that in the early stages after surgery, some people have a hard time digesting the lactose contained in milk. It creates a great deal of gas in their intestines and can be quite uncomfortable. If you are having a tough time with gas, switch the milk in the recipes to vanilla soy milk or water, and you will find little difference in texture or taste. Check to make sure that the soy milk that you choose has plenty of protein; Eden Soy has the most protein per ounce.

If at first you are having a difficult time drinking an entire shake, make a half-recipe of shake, and drink within 30 minutes. The makers of these supplements explain that the protein begins to break down upon contact with water and you will not be getting the full benefit from your efforts. Always make fresh shakes.

When I was planning my plastic surgery I was still drinking my shake every morning to make sure I was getting enough protein. When I am on the run and don't have time to eat during a busy day, I grab a protein bar from my stash in the glove compartment of my car or make myself a protein shake once I get home. I almost always keep a carton of ready-to-drink EAS Carb Control Shakes in the refrigerator so I can grab one on my way out the door if I don't have time to make myself a healthy meal.

I have my entire family drinking protein shakes. Even the average person who has not had weight-loss surgery does not get enough protein—these shakes are an excellent way to give yourself a boost of energy and keep your body strong.

protein shake pantry ingredients

Frozen fresh banana chunks

Frozen fresh papaya cubes

Frozen fresh mango cubes

Frozen unsweetened pineapple cubes

Frozen blueberries, no sugar added

Frozen strawberries, no sugar added

Frozen cherries, no sugar added

Coconut, maple, vanilla, and almond extracts (use pure and natural extracts)

Ground cinnamon

Whole nutmeg

Good quality unsweetened cocoa powder (Droste, Ghirardelli, or Scharffen Berger)

Whipped peanut butter

Instant espresso powder

Da Vinci Sugar Free (SF) Hazelnut, Vanilla, and Strawberry Syrups

frozen banana chunks

Ripe bananas

All the bananas in a bunch obtain perfect ripeness at once, making it obviously impossible to use them before they rot. Peel the bananas, cut each one into 2-inch pieces, and individually wrap each chunk in plastic wrap. Store the banana pieces in a freezer bag and use as desired for protein shakes. One frozen banana chunk in my chocolate shakes makes it creamier.

frozen papaya or mango cubes

Fresh ripe papaya or mango

Peel and seed a perfectly ripe fruit; cut into two-inch cubes and individually wrap in plastic wrap. Store in a freezer bag and use straight from the freezer for tropical protein shakes.

frozen pineapple cubes

One can Dole Pineapple, crushed, in natural juice

Put about one tablespoon crushed pineapple and juice into each section of a plastic ice cube tray. Freeze, then pop out the cubes and store in a freezer bag. Use as a flavoring for tropical protein shakes.

basic shake formula

If at first you cannot drink an entire shake in one sitting, make two smaller shakes, using half of the ingredients, to drink at different times during your day.

½ cup skim milk, soy milk, or water
2 scoops Zero Carb Isopure Creamy Vanilla
About 1 cup ice cubes
Flavoring ingredients, optional

Measure the milk and protein powder into the blender. Add the ice cubes along with the flavoring ingredients you have chosen and quickly pulse the blender on and off until the shake is well-blended, creamy, and frosty. Do not add more liquid; the ice will liquefy to produce a smooth consistency.

Incredible Shake Variations to add to the Basic Shake Formula

vermont banana

> 1 banana chunk
> 1 teaspoon maple extract

cookies and cream

> 2 sugar-free chocolate cream-filled sandwich cookies
>   (Murray is a very good brand)
> 1 heaping tablespoon Cool Whip
> ½ teaspoon vanilla extract

elvis's favorite

> 1 banana chunk
> 1 heaping tablespoon whipped peanut butter
> ½ teaspoon vanilla extract

creamy banana

> 1 banana chunk
> ¼ teaspoon cinnamon
> ½ teaspoon vanilla extract

banana nog

> 1 banana chunk
> ⅛ teaspoon freshly grated nutmeg
> ½ teaspoon vanilla extract

orange–banana frosted

Replace milk in Basic Shake with ¼ cup water
1 banana chunk
¼ cup orange juice
½ teaspoon vanilla extract

chocolate-covered banana

1 banana chunk
2 teaspoons cocoa powder
½ teaspoon vanilla extract

banana bread

1 banana chunk
2 tablespoons SF Hazelnut Syrup

mochaccino

½ teaspoon instant espresso
2 teaspoons cocoa powder
½ teaspoon vanilla extract

grande sugar-free hazelnut latte

1 teaspoon instant espresso
2 tablespoons SF Hazelnut Syrup
Pinch of cinnamon

café méxico

    1 teaspoon instant espresso
    ¼ teaspoon cinnamon

mexican chocolate

    2 teaspoons cocoa powder
    ½ teaspoon vanilla extract
    ¼ teaspoon cinnamon

apple crisp

    ¼ cup no-sugar-added applesauce
    ½ teaspoon cinnamon
    1 tablespoon SF Hazelnut Syrup

peanut butter cup

    2 teaspoons cocoa powder
    1 heaping tablespoon whipped peanut butter
    ½ teaspoon vanilla extract

chocolate cherry

    2 teaspoons cocoa powder
    ¼ cup frozen cherries
    ½ teaspoon almond extract

coconut patty

> **2 teaspoons cocoa powder**
> **1 teaspoon coconut extract**
> **½ teaspoon vanilla extract**

tropical dream

> **2 papaya cubes**
> **1 banana chunk**
> **1 teaspoon coconut extract**
> **½ teaspoon vanilla extract**

pina colada

> **2 pineapple cubes**
> **½ teaspoon coconut extract**
> **½ teaspoon vanilla extract**

cancun sunset

> **1 pineapple cube**
> **3 frozen strawberries**
> **½ teaspoon vanilla extract**

cherry pie

> **¼ cup frozen cherries**
> **½ teaspoon almond extract**
> **½ teaspoon vanilla extract**

soups, purees, and other soft foods

The first real foods eaten after returning home from the hospital are liquids and purees, followed by soft foods. Surgeons vary as to how long we should eat in each category but even a week seems an eternity unless you've planned ahead for some variety. It was easier right from the start to make foods that my whole family could enjoy, instead of preparing separate meals, and I decided that soups would be easiest. When you have a soothing cup of black bean soup to sip, you won't be pressing yourself to move on to the next stage. I made a pot of potato soup and served it to my husband with a salad and crusty loaf of French bread my first week home after surgery. For the first two to three weeks we don't need to be as concerned with carbohydrate counts due to the small amounts we are consuming, so don't let the potato soup worry you. I was happy just sipping my delicious soup, and he marveled that I was eating with him ten days after gastric bypass surgery. I served small ramekins of sugar-free vanilla pudding for dessert with a dollop of Splenda-sweetened whipped cream. It was a major victory for me both physically and in spirit.

A large egg has 7 grams of protein and less than one gram of carbo-hydrates. For the first six months after my surgery, I couldn't stand the texture of hard-cooked egg, so I used eggs in custards, tarts, and omelets to sneak in a few extra grams of soft protein. I enjoyed a Vanilla Egg Custard almost every day for the first three months after my surgery. If you are having a difficult time or are just nervous about eating solid foods for a while, try this custard.

My snacks of mozzarella string cheese were a lifesaver. Who would think that a little one-ounce stick of cheese could be so satisfying? As long as we select lower fat varieties, cheese is a great addition to our diets.

I began eating salads along with soft foods within three to four weeks of my surgery. Adding a few tender leaves of baby lettuce with my tuna and shrimp purees satisfied my craving for vegetables. It is better to dress the entire bowl of greens rather than adding the dressing to individual servings. You use much less dressing, and you get better coverage when you toss the greens in a big bowl. This makes the greens very moist and easy to eat.

As you recuperate and progress, new foods may not always agree with you the first time you try them. If something doesn't go down well, try it again in a few days. I still make the shrimp, salmon, and tuna salad/purees in this section, because they are delicious and provide an excellent protein lunch. I just leave them chunkier now and place a scoop on a bed of baby greens tossed with a little raspberry vinaigrette.

Remember that for the most part the serving counts given are for people who haven't had gastric bypass surgery. When a recipe serves 4, consider that a weight loss surgery or WLS ½ portion is approximately one half of a regular portion except where noted and the nutritional counts are based on the smaller serving that is applicable to us.

stracciatella

WLS ½-cup portion: Calories 34, fat 2 gr, carbs <1 gr,
protein 3.5 gr
Makes 6 cups

Soothing first food when you return home from the hospital.
Make the homemade chicken stock base, and canned soup will
never taste the same again. So many people do not know how to

make chicken soup; if you are one of them, please give it a try for this recipe. Make the stock before you have your surgery and freeze it. When you are home, bring it to a boil and whisk in the remaining ingredients.

6 cups homemade chicken stock (recipe follows)
3 large eggs
¼ cup freshly grated Parmesan
1 tablespoon finely chopped flat-leaf parsley
Pinch of freshly grated nutmeg
Kosher salt and freshly ground black pepper

Bring the stock to a boil in a large saucepan, then reduce the heat and simmer. In a large bowl, beat the eggs with the Parmesan, parsley, and nutmeg with a fork. Add the egg mixture to the broth in a steady stream, stirring vigorously with the fork to break up the egg, which will form fine, light flakes. Season with salt and pepper.

Note: If you need to use store-bought chicken or beef broth, Pacific is a good brand; it comes in 1-quart "juice boxes" (aseptic packaging).

chicken stock

WLS ½-cup portion: Calories 40, fat 1.5 gr, carbs 4.0 gr, protein 3.0 gr
Makes about 4 quarts

After you have enjoyed the soup, use the chicken to make a basic chicken salad, a perfect puree protein food. Remove the tender meat from the chicken once it has cooled and chop it very finely. Don't use the food processor for your chicken salads; it will make an unpalatable chicken paste. Moisten it with a little mayonnaise and a tablespoon of your favorite bottled salad dressing (read the label and make sure the dressing of your choice has less than a gram or two of sugar and carbohydrates). You are looking for a soft consistency as a recent post-op, so add a few spoonfuls of chicken broth from the pot to further moisten the salad.

1 whole 2½- to 3-pound chicken
3 carrots, cut in half
3 celery stalks, cut in half
1 large onion, quartered
2 teaspoons kosher salt
½ teaspoon whole peppercorns

Place all the ingredients in an 8- to 10-quart stockpot and fill with cold water to cover. Bring to a boil, then reduce the heat and simmer, skimming any foam as necessary, for 3½ to 4 hours, until reduced by about one-third. Carefully transfer the chicken to a bowl and pour the stock though a fine mesh sieve set over a large bowl or pot, pressing on the solids to extract as much liquid as possible. Cool the stock at room temperature. Cover and chill until the fat has solidified, at least overnight and up to 3 days. Scrape off and discard the fat.

cream of potato soup

WLS ½-cup portion: Calories 52, fat <1 gr, carbs 9.5 gr, protein 3.5 gr
Makes 6 cups

An excellent first post-op food. An immersion blender allows you to make a smooth soup or sauce right in the pot. If you are within days of your surgery, you will be consuming about ½ cup of soup, so note that the carbohydrate count is calculated accordingly.

3½ cups diced Yukon gold potatoes, peeled, about 1½ pounds or
   4 medium potatoes
½ small onion, chopped
1 medium shallot, sliced
1 quart Chicken Stock (page 104) or low-sodium chicken broth
¼ teaspoon dried thyme
Kosher salt and freshly ground black pepper
½ cup 1% low-fat milk
Shredded Cheddar

Combine the potatoes, onion, shallot, stock, thyme, ½ teaspoon salt, and a few grinds of black pepper in a medium saucepan. Bring to a boil, reduce the heat, and simmer for 15 to 20 minutes, until the potatoes are fork tender. Puree the potato-stock mixture with an immersion blender or in a blender until smooth and creamy. Be careful when pureeing hot liquids in a blender as the steam expands; always cover the lid with a kitchen towel, pulse the switch, then release the steam before proceeding.

Reheat just before serving; add the milk and season with salt and pepper. Top each serving with 1 tablespoon of shredded Cheddar.

creamy black bean soup

WLS ½-cup portion: Calories 62, fat 2.5 gr, carbs 7.5 gr, protein 3.5 gr
Makes 6 cups

Very good

The smooth hot soup will be comforting to both you and your family. A tossed salad and a plate of Cheddar quesadillas with pickled jalapeños round out the meal. This thin but flavorful soup was created for use early after surgery; later on you can add a second can of black beans for a heartier version.

1 tablespoon olive oil

1 small onion, chopped

2 garlic cloves, chopped

One 15-ounce can black beans, rinsed and drained

3 cups Chicken Stock (page 104) or low-sodium chicken broth

½ cup mild roasted tomato salsa (see Note below)

Kosher salt and freshly ground black pepper

½ cup reduced-fat sour cream

Shredded Cheddar, chopped cilantro, and sliced green onions
  (scallions)

Heat the oil in a large, heavy saucepan over medium heat. Sauté the onion and garlic until lightly browned, about 4 minutes. Add the beans, stock, and salsa, and season with salt and pepper. Bring the soup to a boil, reduce the heat, and simmer 10 minutes, stirring occasionally, until the flavors blend and the soup thickens slightly. Puree the soup with an immersion blender or in a blender until smooth and creamy. Be careful when pureeing hot liquids in a blender as the steam expands; always cover the lid with a kitchen towel, pulse the switch, then release the steam before proceeding.

Reheat the soup just before serving and whisk in the sour cream. Check the seasonings. Ladle the soup into bowls and garnish with the Cheddar, cilantro, and green onions. Have a bottle of hot sauce on the table and use to taste.

Note: Rick Bayless, chef/owner of Chicago's Topolobampo and Frontera Grill, is the hand behind the Frontera brand of salsas—they are absolutely delicious.

Newman's Own and Goya salsas are also excellent. Watch for added sugar in other brands.

french onion soup

WLS ½-cup portion: Calories 65.5, fat 2.5 gr, carbs 5 gr, protein 2.5 gr
Makes 6 cups

Another basic soup to have in your repertoire while re-learning to eat after surgery. It is very simple to make and enjoyable to sip. Turkey sandwiches on hard rolls with lettuce and tomato complete a family meal. If you are less than two months post-op, you may wish to omit the cheese from your portion, as it may be too difficult to chew into a smooth mouthful.

1 tablespoon salted butter
1 tablespoon olive oil
2 medium white onions, chopped, about 1½ pounds
2 medium red onions, chopped, about 1½ pounds
2 large shallots, chopped
2 garlic cloves, chopped
1 cup white wine
1 quart beef broth (see Note, page 104)
2 cups low-sodium chicken broth
½ teaspoon Tabasco sauce
1 teaspoon Worcestershire sauce
¼ teaspoon freshly grated nutmeg
Kosher salt and freshly ground black pepper
½ cup finely shredded Swiss cheese, about ⅛ pound

Heat the butter and olive oil in a large, heavy pot over medium-low heat. Sauté the onions, shallots, and garlic until very soft and brown, about 30 minutes, stirring frequently. Add the wine and continue to cook until the mixture is reduced to a thick glaze. Stir in the beef broth, chicken broth, Tabasco, Worcestershire, and nutmeg. Reduce the heat and simmer for 45 minutes. Season with salt and pepper.

To serve, reheat the soup to boiling, ladle into bowls, and sprinkle with some of the cheese.

hummus

WLS ¼-cup portion: Calories 65.5, fat 4 gr, carbs 6.4 gr, protein 2 gr
Makes 2 cups

Eating right after surgery can be a chore. It is hard to find foods that are smooth and palatable and have some protein value. I loved homemade hummus before my surgery, so it was a natural to give it a try post-op. I put a small amount in a custard cup and used a pita chip to eat it, nibbling just a tiny bit of the chip at a time. The one or two pita chips gave me a little needed crunch that I craved after an extended period of soft foods and added only minimal carbohydrates to my daily total.

One 16-ounce can chickpeas, rinsed and drained
3 garlic cloves, thinly sliced
⅓ cup tahini (sesame paste)
2 tablespoons fresh lemon juice (about 1 lemon)
2 tablespoons extra-virgin olive oil
Kosher salt and freshly ground black pepper
2 tablespoons coarsely chopped flat-leaf parsley
Toasted pita chips (recipe follows)

In a food processor or blender, puree the chickpeas with the garlic, tahini, lemon juice, olive oil, and as much water as necessary to process the hummus to a smooth mayonnaise consistency, scraping down the sides to incorporate all the chickpeas. Add salt and pepper to taste and transfer to a bowl. Sprinkle with the parsley. Serve with the pita chips.

pita chips

3 pita rounds

Split each pita into 2 rounds; cut each round into 16 pieces. Arrange on a baking sheet and bake at 350°F until lightly browned and crisp, 10 to 12 minutes.

pinto bean dip

WLS ¼-cup portion: Calories 59, fat 2 gr, carbs 8 gr, protein 2.5 gr
Makes 2 cups

Another smooth, easy-to-digest puree. Make turkey burgers or hamburgers on soft sesame seed rolls for the rest of the family, serving this dish as a "refried bean" side dish with a dollop of sour cream, extra cheese, and a few pickled jalapeño slices.

1 tablespoon olive oil
1 small onion, minced
2 garlic cloves, minced
One 16-ounce can pinto beans, rinsed and drained
½ to 1 cup low-sodium chicken broth (see Note, page 104)
¼ teaspoon ground cumin
Kosher salt and freshly ground black pepper
1 tablespoon finely chopped cilantro
½ cup shredded Cheddar, about ¼ pound

Sauté the onion and garlic in the oil in a large nonstick skillet over medium-high heat, stirring constantly until lightly browned and very soft, about 6 minutes. Add the beans and mash with a potato masher or the back of a large wooden spoon to make a coarse puree. Stir in enough broth to thin to a creamy consistency. Continue to cook, stirring occasionally, until the mixture is hot. Add the cumin and season with salt and pepper. Remove from the heat and stir in the cilantro and Cheddar.

shrimp salad spread

WLS ½-cup portion: Calories 115, fat 7 gr, carbs <1 gr, protein 12 gr
Makes 2½ cups

I practically live on this shrimp salad, even two and a half years after my bariatric surgery. It is extremely moist, high in protein, and extraordinarily delicious. I sauté a pound of shrimp, mix it up with the remaining ingredients in my mini food processor and keep it in a bowl in my refrigerator for quick lunches and suppers, or even a snack if I am so inclined. I don't snack often, but I know that a couple of tablespoons of shrimp salad on a melba round is better than a handful of Fritos or crackers, which will destroy my carbohydrate count for the day.

Early after my surgery I pureed this into a smooth shrimp paste, but now I leave it much chunkier and use more Old Bay seasoning to spice it up. I toss a handful of mixed baby greens with a little dressing and put my portion of shrimp salad on top. Sautéing the shrimp in a bit of olive oil rather than poaching or boiling them in water concentrates the flavor of the seafood and gives it another layer of taste.

½ teaspoon olive oil

pound medium shrimp, peeled and deveined

¼ cup light mayonnaise (see Note)

Juice of ½ lemon, about 1 tablespoon

2 green onions (scallions), sliced, including the green tops

1 teaspoon Old Bay Seasoning

Heat the olive oil in a large nonstick skillet over medium-high heat. Add the shrimp and sauté for 2 to 3 minutes, stirring constantly, until just opaque throughout. Transfer to a small bowl and set aside. Blend the mayonnaise, lemon juice, green onions, and Old Bay Seasoning in a food processor until smooth; add the shrimp and pulse until they are very finely chopped and the mixture is well blended. Transfer to a serving bowl, cover, and chill.

Note: I prefer Hellmann's Mayonnaise (Best Foods in the western U.S.). They make regular, light, and reduced-fat versions.

mediterranean tuna spread

WLS ½ cup portion: Calories 85, fat 3.5 gr, carbs <1 gr, protein 11 gr
Makes 2½ cups

Tuna is another mainstay of my diet! The new pouches of tuna have a fresh taste and are so much more flavorful than the canned variety; give them a try. Since they are packed without the addition of water, I add a little chicken broth or water for a moister consistency.

Two 6-ounce pouches albacore tuna

2 tablespoons reduced-fat mayonnaise

Juice of 1 lemon, about 2 tablespoons

2 tablespoons drained and finely chopped roasted red peppers

**10 Kalamata or oil-cured olives, pitted and finely chopped
   (see Note below)**

2 tablespoons finely minced red onion

Kosher salt and freshly ground black pepper to taste

Empty the tuna into a small bowl and mash with a fork until very finely flaked. Add the mayonnaise, lemon juice, roasted peppers, olives, and onion and stir to combine, adding a little water or chicken broth to further moisten. Add salt and pepper to taste.

Note: It is becoming more common to find displays of olives in many markets, and any black olive that appeals to you will work in this recipe. Smash the olives with the flat side of a large knife. The pit will easily come away from the olive.

curried chicken
and almond spread

*WLS ½-cup portion: Calories 113, fat 7 gr, carbs 1 gr,
protein 11 gr*
Makes 2½ cups

I make this salad with the chicken left over from a pot of chicken stock. Transfer the whole chicken to a large bowl, allow it to cool, and remove and discard the bones and the skin. Finely chop the chicken meat with a knife. A food processor will turn the tender meat into a blob of unpalatable chicken paste. This is also a great salad to make with a take-out rotisserie chicken. Serve a small scoop of some dressed baby greens on top.

1½ teaspoons curry powder

2 tablespoons light mayonnaise

2 tablespoons nonfat yogurt

Juice of 1 lemon, about 2 tablespoons

Kosher salt and freshly ground black pepper

2 cups very finely chopped cooked chicken

1 tablespoon minced red onion

1 tablespoon minced fresh flat-leaf parsley

1 tablespoon finely chopped almonds

2 to 3 tablespoons low-sodium chicken broth (see Note, page 104)

Toast the curry powder in a small skillet over medium heat until a wisp of smoke appears and the mixture is fragrant, about 30 seconds. Transfer to a medium bowl and blend with the mayonnaise, yogurt, and lemon juice, and season with salt and pepper. Add the chicken, onion, parsley, and almonds; blend until the mixture is well combined, adding a little broth to moisten further.

salmon salad

WLS ½-cup portion: Calories 91, fat 3.5 gr, carbs 2.5 gr, protein 12.5 gr
Makes 2½ cups

Salmon is high in protein, readily available, and moist and tender to eat. Roast a double portion of salmon for dinner and chill the leftovers to make this salad for the next day's lunch.

1 pound cooked salmon fillet, skin and bones removed, then chilled
3 green onions (scallions), minced
¼ cup bottled Raspberry & Balsamic Dressing (see Note), or
    Sesame Dressing (page 180)
Kosher salt and freshly ground black pepper
Baby spinach, rinsed and dried

Flake the salmon into fine pieces. Add the green onions and salad dressing and gently combine with the salmon mixture. Add salt and pepper to taste. Serve a small portion on top of a bed of lightly dressed baby spinach leaves.

Note: Consorzio is a flavorful brand of Raspberry & Balsamic Dressing that I use regularly (see Sources, page 251).

turkey tomato ragù

WLS ½-cup portion: Calories 107, fat 5.5 gr, carbs 4 gr, protein 11 gr
Serves 4 when used as pasta sauce

Very good

This thick, meaty, chili-type dish is very easy to eat when you first try different pureed and soft foods. If you mash the turkey with a fork while it is browning, you will end up with a very fine-textured mixture to eat by the spoonful. Cook some ziti or bow tie pasta and use the remaining ragù as a sauce for the rest of the family.

1 teaspoon olive oil
1 pound ground turkey breast
1 garlic clove, minced
1 small red onion, minced
One 14-ounce can tomato sauce

2 teaspoons dried basil
½ teaspoon dried oregano
½ teaspoon dried thyme
Kosher salt and freshly ground black pepper

Heat the olive oil in a deep covered skillet over medium-high heat. Brown the turkey, mashing with a wooden spoon or fork to break up chunks. Add the garlic and onion and cook until softened, stirring occasionally. Stir in the tomato sauce and 1 cup water, then add the basil, oregano, and thyme, and season with salt and pepper. Cover and simmer over low heat for 20 minutes, or until the flavors are blended.

Note: I have substituted a high-protein soy crumble product for the turkey and it is nearly indistinguishable.

Variation: This recipe can also go Mexican with the substitution of 2 teaspoons of chili powder for the basil. Serve it in a deep bowl ladled over a scoop of white rice and sprinkled with sliced green onions.

protein pudding treat

*WLS ½-cup portion: Calories 84, fat <1 gr, carbs 6 gr,
protein 20 gr*
Makes 3 cups

When you come home from the hospital you won't have an appetite for anything more than some comforting pudding. I existed on sugar-free pudding and Crystal Light to the extent that I joked that if I knew I could lose this much weight by eliminating everything but these two foods, I would have done it instead of having weight loss surgery. I fortified my pudding with protein powder and came up with a winner. Three cups of pudding contain more than 100 grams of protein.

1 box Jell-O Sugar Free Instant Pudding mix, any flavor

2 cups skim milk, cold

½ teaspoon vanilla, coconut, or almond extract

4 scoops protein powder, such as Zero Carb Isopure Creamy
   Vanilla, or ProPlete Gold Banana Creme (see Sources, page 246)

¾ cup Cool Whip

Pour the dry pudding mix into a medium bowl. Whisk in the milk and vanilla. Mix until smooth and thickened. Whisk in the protein powder and fold in the whipped topping to lighten. Chill the mixture.

vanilla egg custard

WLS ½-cup portion: Calories 110, fat 4.5 gr, carbs 7.5 gr,
protein 9 gr
Makes six ½-cup servings

This custard is smooth, cold, and very soothing. I made a batch at least twice a week, as my family loved this as well. Purchase 6 or 8 four-ounce custard cups; they are invaluable for portion control.

4 large eggs

1 cup skim milk

1½ cups evaporated low-fat milk

½ cup Splenda Granular

2 teaspoons vanilla extract

Pinch of Kosher salt

Freshly grated nutmeg

Preheat the oven to 325°F. Place 6 custard cups or ramekins in a large roasting pan and set aside. Whisk together the eggs, milk, evaporated milk, Splenda, vanilla, and salt. Pour through a fine mesh sieve into a

large measuring cup. Divide evenly among the custard cups and grate
a generous amount of nutmeg over each one. Pour enough hot water in
the roasting pan to come about halfway up the sides of the custard
cups. Bake 25 to 35 minutes, until the custards are just set in the center. Carefully remove the custards from the water bath, and transfer to
a wire rack to cool. Serve chilled.

green chile cheese puff
with roasted tomato salsa

WLS ½ portion: Calories 163, fat 10 gr, carbs 6 gr, protein 12 gr
Serves 4

This dinner is full of protein and flavor, while the roasted salsa
accompaniment makes the soufflé extra moist. While the soufflé-
like puff bakes, I make a salad of mixed baby greens, sliced grape
tomatoes, thin cucumber slices, and red onions, and toss it with
store-bought ranch dressing. A handful of golden baked pita
chips (page 110) rounds out the meal for the family.

roasted tomato salsa

4 large ripe Roma tomatoes, cut in half lengthwise
1 garlic clove, peeled and left whole
1 small red onion, peeled and sliced
1 jalapeño chile, cut in half lengthwise, stemmed, and seeded
Juice of 1 lime, about 1½ tablespoons
1 tablespoon olive oil
2 tablespoons chopped cilantro
Kosher salt and freshly ground black pepper

Green chile cheese puff

> **Vegetable oil cooking spray**
> **¼ cup all-purpose flour**
> **¾ teaspoon kosher salt**
> **½ teaspoon baking powder**
> **6 large eggs**
> **2 tablespoons salted butter, melted**
> **1 cup 2% low-fat cottage cheese**
> **1 cup freshly shredded medium-sharp Cheddar cheese,**
>   **about ¼ pound**
> **Two 4-ounce cans diced mild green chiles, drained**
> **Roasted tomato salsa**

Preheat the broiler to the highest temperature. Line a baking sheet with foil, folding up the edges to catch the juices. Arrange the tomatoes, garlic, onion slices, and jalapeño on the baking sheet and broil for 8 minutes, or until the vegetables are lightly charred and softened. Lift the foil, being careful to keep the juices, and pour into a blender or food processor. Add the lime juice, olive oil, and cilantro, and pulse the mixture until it is an even consistency but not completely smooth. Season with salt and pepper to taste and set aside.

Preheat the oven to 350°F. Lightly coat a 9-inch glass pie plate with cooking spray. Sift together the flour, salt, and baking powder into a small bowl and set aside. Beat the eggs in a large bowl with an electric mixer until doubled in volume, about 4 minutes. Blend in the flour mixture and melted butter. Stir in the cottage cheese, Cheddar, and green chiles. Pour the mixture into the prepared pie plate. Bake the custard in the middle of the oven for 30 to 40 minutes, until the top is puffed and golden brown and a sharp knife inserted near the center comes out clean. Cut the cheese puff into wedges and spoon some of the roasted tomato salsa over each piece.

sunday morning frittata

WLS ½ portion: Calories 130, fat 8 gr, carbs 4 gr, protein 11 gr
Serves 4

Packed with protein and soft enough to eat very early in your
post-op period. Be creative with your choice of vegetables and
cheese, keeping track of the carbohydrate count. Serve for
breakfast with a fresh melon or a berry compote, or for supper
with a tossed salad.

1 tablespoon salted butter
1 small zucchini, finely diced
8 mushrooms, finely diced
6 large eggs
½ cup 1% low-fat milk
1 cup 2% low-fat cottage cheese
1 cup shredded Jarlsberg or Swiss cheese, about ¼ pound
3 green onions (scallions), sliced
1 ripe Roma tomato, diced
1 tablespoon chopped fresh dill
Vegetable oil cooking spray

Preheat the oven to 350°F. Heat the butter in a medium nonstick skillet and lightly sauté the zucchini and mushrooms until the released
juices have reduced and the vegetables are lightly browned. In a large
bowl, beat the eggs with the milk until well blended, then stir in the
cottage cheese, Jarlsberg cheese, green onions, tomato, dill, and the
sautéed vegetables. Pour into a 9 × 9-inch baking dish that has been
lightly coated with cooking spray. Bake for 40 to 45 minutes, until a
knife inserted near the center comes out clean.

If using 4 individual ramekins, place them on a baking sheet and bake for 25 to 30 minutes, until still a bit soft in the center.

mexican meatball soup

WLS ½-cup portion: Calories 79, fat 4 gr, carbs 5.5 gr, protein 5.5 gr
Makes six 1-cup servings

This soup works at all post-op food stages. In the early stages, eat a couple of the tiny meatballs for a little protein. I serve my family some quesadilla wedges made with pepper Jack cheese and a bowl of homemade guacamole.

1 tablespoon olive oil
1 large sweet onion, finely diced
4 garlic cloves, minced
1 bay leaf
1 quart Chicken Stock (page 104) or canned low-sodium broth
One 16-ounce can diced tomatoes (see Note)
½ cup medium-hot tomato salsa (see Note, page 107)
¾ cup chopped fresh cilantro
½ pound ground turkey breast
2 tablespoons minced red onion
2 tablespoons yellow cornmeal
3 tablespoons skim milk
1 large egg
¼ teaspoon ground cumin
Kosher salt and freshly ground black pepper
Tabasco sauce to taste

Heat the oil in large covered pot over medium high heat. Add the onion, half of the garlic, and the bay leaf and sauté until very soft and golden brown, about 8 minutes. Add the broth, tomatoes with juice, salsa, and about one-third of the cilantro. Bring to a boil, then cover, reduce the heat, and simmer for 15 minutes.

Combine the turkey, red onion, cornmeal, milk, egg, cumin, ½ teaspoon salt, a few grinds of black pepper, the remaining garlic, and another third of the cilantro, blending well. Shape the meat by rolling generous tablespoons into 1-inch balls. Add the meatballs to the soup and bring to a low boil, stirring occasionally. Cover the soup, reduce the heat, and simmer 20 minutes. Season with salt, pepper, and Tabasco; stir in the remaining cilantro.

Note: If you can find Muir Glen Fire Roasted Tomatoes, use them in this soup. They are also excellent for many other recipes in this book.

light manicotti

WLS portion of ½ manicotti: Calories 96, fat 4.5 gr, carbs 6.6 gr, protein 7 gr
Makes 10 pieces of manicotti

Italian comfort food that is also very soft and easy to eat. I don't eat pasta anymore; it has too many carbohydrates and gives me an uncomfortably full feeling even in small amounts, but I do enjoy these tender, cheese-filled egg crepes. I make this dish for Sunday dinner and everyone is happy. You can use the Italian Meatballs recipe on page 189 to add to the sauce for this recipe. Serve your manicotti with a tossed salad dressed with balsamic vinegar and olive oil along with a loaf of Italian bread.

sauce

1 tablespoon olive oil

1 small onion, diced

2 garlic cloves, minced

One 28-ounce can crushed Italian tomatoes

One 4-ounce can tomato paste

1 tablespoon dried basil

½ teaspoon dried oregano

½ teaspoon dried thyme

¼ teaspoon crushed red pepper

Kosher salt and freshly ground black pepper

crepes

1 cup all-purpose flour

½ cup 1% milk

3 large eggs

½ teaspoon kosher salt

Olive oil or vegetable cooking spray

filling

1 pound part skim milk ricotta

½ cup shredded part skim milk mozzarella, plus additional for
   topping

¼ cup freshly grated Parmesan

2 large eggs

3 tablespoons chopped flat-leaf parsley

Heat the olive oil in a large saucepan over medium-high heat. Sauté the onion and garlic until softened. Add the tomatoes, tomato paste, and 1 cup water. Stir in the basil, oregano, thyme, and red pepper, season with salt and pepper, bring the sauce to a boil, then reduce the heat and simmer while preparing the crepes and filling.

In a large bowl, blend the flour, milk, eggs, and salt until smooth. Heat an 8-inch nonstick skillet over medium heat and lightly grease with a few drops of olive oil or cooking spray. Ladle 2 tablespoons of the batter into the center of the pan. Lift the pan from the burner and swirl it so the batter smoothly coats the entire bottom. Replace the pan on the burner and cook just until the surface looks dry. Using a spatula or your fingers, flip the crepe and cook a few seconds until the other side is lightly browned. Repeat with the remaining batter to make 10 crepes.

Preheat the oven to 375°F. Blend the ricotta, mozzarella, and Parmesan with the eggs and parsley. Spoon the filling into a large plastic bag, squeeze out the air, and snip about ½ inch off of one corner. Spread 1 cup of the tomato sauce on the bottom of a large shallow baking dish. Lay a crepe on a flat surface, pipe about ¼ cup of the filling in a thick line down the center by squeezing the bag, then roll the crepe, tucking in the sides. Place the rolled crepe in the prepared baking dish, seam side down. Repeat with the remaining crepes. Cover the crepes with tomato sauce, sprinkle with mozzarella, and bake for 40 minutes, or until hot and bubbling.

fish and seafood

Most post-op weight loss surgery people will tell you that seafood is the perfect food for them to eat because of the soft, moist texture, high protein, and low fat content. Fish contains about 7 grams of protein per ounce, so a 5-ounce serving of broiled grouper has 35 grams of protein! Top that with charred tomato vinaigrette to further moisten the fish and you have a dinner that's suitable even for guests.

I have always loved seafood so it has been easy for me to leave the sirloin behind and concentrate on shrimp and swordfish. If you can't find the particular fish suggested in the recipe, substitute one with a similar texture. A large percentage of WLS people have never cooked seafood because its purchase and preparation intimidate many novice cooks. If you follow a few basic guidelines, you will be able to prepare many of these recipes in less than 30 minutes.

Smell is the key indicator of freshness. Fresh fish has a clean, bright, fresh smell. Don't buy it if it has a "fishy" or ammonia odor. I usually buy my fish in a specialty fish market where I have a better guarantee of quality. Once the folks behind the counter get to know you, they will recommend what just came in, or guide you to which catch is of exceptional quality. I popped into my local fish market yesterday and the man at the counter was very excited about the wild white salmon that had just come in from Alaska. He asked me if I liked sushi, and when I told him that I loved it, he grabbed a huge fillet from the ice, cut a beautiful paper-thin sashimi slice, and we shared a treat. The unadorned slice of fish was meaty and clean tasting, with a touch of salt from the sea. I left the store with a nice fillet for our supper tucked into a bag with ice.

The secret to moist fish is to not overcook it. The general rule of thumb is to cook fish 8 to 10 minutes per inch of thickness, measuring the fillet or steak at its thickest point. So, a salmon fillet approximately one inch thick should be cooked for no more than 8 to 10 minutes total. Sauté a much thinner ¼-inch flounder fillet for only 2 to 3 minutes. I keep a ruler in my kitchen gadget drawer to help estimate cooking times.

We can also rely on seafood when eating in restaurants. I no longer hesitate when faced with an impromptu lunch or dinner situation. I know I can find a protein source that works for me, such as a salmon Caesar salad, tuna melt, or shrimp cocktail, on any menu. When ordering from a menu you have to think about what the texture will be when you chew a bite of the food; a bite of grilled salmon with mango salsa will always be moister than a bite of roasted chicken breast.

Several of my first restaurant meals when I was 6 to 8 weeks post-op were at our favorite sushi bar. I was a bit nervous but with a little thought I was able to put together a perfect sushi dinner. I picked apart some of the rolls, ate only the fish from my sushi, and had a very successful first outing. Since my sushi chef noticed that I was leaving the rice and the seaweed wrappers, he has created a roll for me that is perfect for WLS sushi lovers. The nori wrappers were too tough for me to chew really well at first, so he made a small roll using a sheet of moistened rice paper, with chopped spicy tuna, avocado slices, scallions, and a spicy Japanese mayonnaise dipping sauce. He also prepared raw tuna and yellowtail for me sashimi-style in paper-thin slices that I dip in ponzu sauce. Everything is very tender, easy to chew, and tastes great. I do not eat rice, since it is too high in carbohydrates and would fill me up before I got to my protein.

These seafood recipes serve four people who have not had gastric bypass surgery. The person who is eating after having had bypass surgery would be eating about one half of one serving. For example, a recipe using 1½ pounds of shrimp would feed 4 people with a 6-ounce portion per person; the WLS ½ portion would be a 3-ounce portion with enough of the sauce to moisten it. The nutritional analysis has been calculated for the WLS ½ portion including the sauce or salsa for that dish.

mykonos shrimp with feta

WLS ½ portion: Calories 207, fat 10 gr, carbs 8 gr, protein 18 gr
Serves 4

Shrimp are incredibly moist, making them texturally one of the easiest proteins to eat after surgery. They are my favorite food! I keep bags of raw, flash-frozen, peeled and deveined shrimp in the freezer, so this is a quick meal to prepare when I'm running late. I thaw the frozen shrimp in a bowl of cool water and by the time the remaining ingredients are prepared, the shrimp will be defrosted.

When I make this dish for a special occasion, I use individual, hand-painted baking dishes that can go under the broiler so each guest gets their own portion. A salad of baby spinach leaves tossed with oil-cured olives and red onions, dressed with a little lemon juice and olive oil, completes this meal.

3 tablespoons olive oil
1 large onion, thinly sliced
3 garlic cloves, thinly sliced
One 14-ounce can diced tomatoes, drained (see Note, page 122)
½ cup white wine
1 teaspoon dried oregano
⅛ teaspoon ground cinnamon
Kosher salt and freshly ground black pepper

½ cup chopped flat-leaf parsley

1½ pounds large shrimp, peeled and deveined

2 medium tomatoes, peeled with a vegetable peeler then
    thinly sliced

¼ pound Greek feta cheese, rinsed, drained, and crumbled

Preheat the oven to 450°F. Sauté the onion and garlic in 1 tablespoon of the olive oil in a nonstick skillet over medium-high heat until golden brown. Add the diced tomatoes, wine, oregano, and cinnamon; lightly season with salt and pepper and cook until most of the liquid has evaporated, about 12 minutes. Stir in half of the parsley and spoon the sauce evenly over the bottom of a decorative baking dish. Sauté the shrimp in 1 tablespoon of the olive oil in a nonstick skillet over high heat until they just begin to turn pink and curl, about 2 minutes. Arrange the shrimp on top of the sauce in the baking dish, add a layer of the sliced tomatoes and then the feta; drizzle with the remaining olive oil and a few grinds of black pepper. Bake 15 to 18 minutes, until the sauce is bubbling. Turn the broiler to high and cook an additional 1 to 2 minutes, until the feta is golden. Garnish with the remaining parsley and serve immediately.

bengal shrimp korma

WLS ½ portion: Calories 103, fat 3 gr, carbs 3 gr, protein 15 gr
Serves 4

This Indian combination can be thrown together in minutes if you have the seasonings on hand. My family enjoys it with steamed rice and sautéed broccoli. I have simmered sea scallops and even a large whole grouper fillet in this flavorful sauce with spectacular results.

3 tablespoons nonfat yogurt

1 teaspoon sweet paprika

1 teaspoon garam masala (see Notes)

1 tablespoon tomato paste

½ cup light coconut milk

½ teaspoon chili powder

Kosher salt

1 tablespoon peanut oil

2 garlic cloves, minced

1 teaspoon grated fresh ginger

¼ teaspoon ground cinnamon

1 teaspoon cornstarch dissolved in 1 tablespoon coconut milk

1½ pounds large shrimp, peeled and deveined

2 tablespoons coarsely chopped cilantro

Freshly ground black pepper

Whisk together the yogurt, paprika, garam masala, tomato paste, coconut milk, chili powder, and ⅔ cup water in a small bowl, season with ½ teaspoon salt, and set aside. Heat the peanut oil in a deep nonstick skillet over medium heat and sauté the garlic, ginger, and cinnamon for 1 to 2 minutes, until fragrant. Add the yogurt mixture and bring to a boil, stirring occasionally, then lower the heat and simmer 5 minutes to blend the flavors. Stir in the cornstarch mixture and cook until thick and smooth. Add the shrimp and simmer, until the shrimp start to curl and are just cooked through, 2 to 3 minutes. Stir in the cilantro and season with salt and pepper.

Notes: Garam masala is an Indian spice blend that may include black pepper, cardamom, cinnamon, cumin, and cloves.

Either the same day or the next day, I usually make the coconut custards (page 204) for dessert to use the remaining coconut milk from this recipe.

grilled shrimp
with romesco sauce

WLS ½ portion: Calories 149, fat 8 gr, carbs 3 gr, protein 16 gr
Serves 4

Creamy red pepper aioli—in this Spanish version with almonds, called *romesco*—is delicious with all types of grilled or roasted fish and chicken. This recipe makes about one cup of sauce, which is plenty for two meals. Pair the leftover sauce with grilled chicken thighs. Serve with roasted asparagus and a tomato salad dressed with balsamic vinegar and olive oil.

4 garlic cloves
½ medium onion, cut into ½-inch slices
¼ cup whole almonds
One 1-inch slice French bread, cubed
1 Roma tomato, cut in half lengthwise
3 tablespoons olive oil
¼ cup roasted red peppers, drained well and patted dry
1 tablespoon red wine vinegar
¼ teaspoon crushed red pepper
1 teaspoon sweet paprika
Kosher salt and freshly ground black pepper
1½ pounds jumbo shrimp, peeled and butterflied

Preheat the oven to 400°F. Arrange the garlic, onion, almonds, bread, and tomatoes on a baking sheet, drizzle with 1 teaspoon of the olive oil, and roast for 12 to 15 minutes, until the vegetables are softened and the bread and almonds are golden. Transfer to a food processor and add the roasted peppers, vinegar, red pepper, and paprika. Pulse until well combined, then slowly add the remaining olive oil, blending until the sauce is smooth and creamy. Season with salt and pepper.

Arrange the shrimp on small bamboo skewers and sear in a non-stick skillet or grill pan over high heat for 3 to 4 minutes, until just opaque throughout. Spoon a little of the sauce on each plate and arrange the shrimp around the sauce.

shrimp with roasted
red onion and tomatillo salsa

WLS ½ portion: Calories 128, fat 5 gr, carbs 5 gr, protein 15 gr
Serves 4

Tomatillos look like green tomatoes, but they are related to the gooseberry. Popular in Latin-American cooking, tomatillos are the main ingredient in many green salsas or roasted salsa verde, lending a refreshing tartness. If you have never tasted them, give this recipe a try—they blend beautifully with the roasted red onion, jalapeños, garlic, and touch of lime.

12 medium fresh tomatillos, husks removed, rinsed, and
   halved
2 fresh jalapeño chiles, halved lengthwise, stemmed, and seeded
4 garlic cloves
1 small red onion, cut into ½-inch slices
2 tablespoons olive oil
Kosher salt
2 tablespoons coarsely chopped fresh cilantro
Juice of 1 lime, 1½ to 2 tablespoons
Freshly ground black pepper
1½ pounds large shrimp, peeled and deveined

Preheat the broiler. Arrange the tomatillos and jalapeños cut side down along with the garlic and onion slices on a baking sheet; drizzle with 1 tablespoon of the olive oil and sprinkle lightly with salt. Broil until the vegetables are charred on top and very soft, about 15 minutes. Empty the softened vegetables and any liquid into a food processor; pulse until chunky; add the cilantro and process to a coarse puree. Transfer to a medium bowl, stir in the lime juice, and season with salt and pepper.

Heat the remaining tablespoon of olive oil over medium-high heat in a nonstick skillet and sauté the shrimp until they begin to turn pink. Add enough of the roasted red onion and tomatillo sauce to generously coat, and cook until the shrimp are just cooked through and the sauce is bubbling, about 4 minutes.

shrimp creole

WLS ½ portion: Calories 117, fat 3 gr, carbs 7 gr, protein 15 gr
Serves 4

The traditional Louisiana favorite, a flavorful "trinity" of vegetables simmered in a tomato base and spiced up with Worcestershire, Tabasco, and a home-blended Creole seasoning. Use the biggest shrimp you can find and poach them in this delicious sauce just until they have firmed up and are opaque in the center. Serve the shrimp with a ladle of sauce over some steamed rice for those who are not watching their carbohydrate count, and sautéed zucchini as a side dish.

1 tablespoon olive oil
½ cup chopped onions
½ cup chopped celery
½ cup diced green bell peppers
2 garlic cloves, chopped

One 16-ounce can diced tomatoes with juice

One 8-ounce can tomato sauce

1 tablespoon Worcestershire sauce

1 teaspoon Creole Seasoning Blend (recipe follows) or prepared
   Cajun or Creole blend

2 teaspoons Tabasco sauce, plus additional to taste

1 teaspoon cornstarch

Kosher salt and freshly ground black pepper

1½ pounds large shrimp, peeled and deveined

Sauté the onions, celery, peppers, and garlic in the olive oil in a covered nonstick skillet over medium heat until the vegetables are softened. Add the tomatoes, tomato sauce, Worcestershire, Creole Seasoning, and Tabasco. Cover the pan, reduce the heat, and simmer 45 minutes, until the vegetables are tender. Blend the cornstarch with 1 tablespoon water, stir into the sauce, and cook until the mixture thickens. Season with salt, pepper, and additional Tabasco to taste. Add the shrimp, cover, and simmer 4 to 5 minutes, until the shrimp are pink and just cooked through.

creole seasoning blend

2½ tablespoons sweet paprika

2 tablespoons kosher salt

2 tablespoons garlic powder

1 tablespoon black pepper

1 tablespoon onion powder

1 tablespoon cayenne

1 tablespoon dried oregano

1 tablespoon dried thyme

Combine all ingredients thoroughly and store in an airtight jar or container.

Note: If you'd rather use a prepared blend, Tony Chachere's makes several excellent Creole seasonings (see Sources, page 252).

shrimp ceviche

*WLS ½ portion: Calories 166, fat 9 gr, carbs 6.5 gr,
protein 15.5 gr
Serves 4*

When I lived in Mexico, nothing was tastier on a sunny afternoon
than a ceviche cocktail mixto, prepared with chunks of fresh
snapper, conch, and shrimp, all "cooked" by the acid in the lime
juice and tossed with tomatoes, onion, cilantro, and a touch of
habanero. The little open-air seafood restaurants along the beach
served these delicious salads piled in old-fashioned ice cream
sundae glasses with half of a lime and a basket of freshly fried
tortilla chips. Here, the shrimp are briefly poached to make them
tender.

Kosher salt and freshly ground black pepper
Juice of 4 limes (about ¾ cup), plus 1 lime cut into
   wedges
1¼ pounds medium shrimp, peeled and deveined
3 ripe Roma tomatoes, diced
1 small red onion, finely diced
1 jalapeño chile, stemmed, seeded, and very finely
   minced
½ cup green olive pieces
½ cup roughly chopped cilantro
2 tablespoons olive oil
1 tablespoon ketchup
Tabasco sauce to taste
4 corn tortillas
1 small ripe Hass avocado, peeled and cut into 1-inch
   cubes

Fill a large saucepan halfway with water, add 1 tablespoon salt, the juice and rind of 1 lime (about 1½ tablespoons of juice), and bring to a boil over high heat. Add the shrimp, remove from the heat, and poach for 60 to 90 seconds. Drain the shrimp and then immediately rinse with cool water. Peel and devein the poached shrimp and place in a large bowl. Add the tomatoes, onion, jalapeño, olives, cilantro, olive oil, ketchup, lime juice, and Tabasco and combine to blend. Season with salt and pepper. Chill before serving.

Preheat the oven to 350°F. Cut the tortillas into eighths and spread out on a baking sheet; sprinkle with salt and bake 10 to 15 minutes, until golden and crisp.

Serve a generous portion of the ceviche in a martini glass or decorative dish, garnishing with a few avocado cubes, a lime wedge, and baked tortilla chips.

Note: Avocados are ripe when they are almost black and yield slightly when pressed with your thumb.

southern shrimp and grits

WLS ½ portion: Calories 133, fat 6 gr, carbs 3 gr, protein 16 gr
Serves 4

This version of the low country favorite is spicy, but you can tame it if you would like by cutting the seasoning in half and using less Tabasco. I buy my stone-ground grits from a mill in northern Georgia. My husband and his family can't believe an Italian from New Jersey can make such a delicious bowl of grits. I have my shrimp and sauce in a bowl and pass on the grits. The WLS portion does not include any grits in the nutritional analysis.

1¼ pounds large shrimp, peeled and deveined

1 teaspoon Creole Seasoning Blend, page 133, or prepared
   Creole or Cajun blend (see Note, page 133)

1½ teaspoons sweet paprika

Juice of 1 lemon, about 2 tablespoons

Kosher salt

1 cup stone-ground white grits (see Note)

1 tablespoon salted butter

½ cup shredded Cheddar, about ⅛ pound

2 teaspoons Tabasco sauce

Freshly ground black pepper

3 slices bacon, cut into 1-inch pieces

1 small onion, chopped

3 garlic cloves, thinly sliced

½ cup chopped green bell pepper

½ cup low-sodium chicken broth

2 teaspoons Worcestershire sauce

1 teaspoon cornstarch

4 green onions (scallions), thinly sliced

Toss the shrimp with the Creole seasoning, paprika, and lemon juice in a large bowl until evenly coated. Set aside.

Prepare the grits in a large heavy saucepan, first bringing 3 cups of water and 1 teaspoon of salt to a boil. Slowly whisk in the grits, cover, and reduce the heat to a very low simmer. Cook, stirring occasionally, for 25 to 30 minutes, until the grits are thick and creamy. Stir in the butter, cheese, and 1 teaspoon of Tabasco, and season with salt and pepper. Set aside.

Brown the bacon in a nonstick skillet over medium-high heat and transfer to a paper towel to drain. Add the onion, garlic, and green pepper to the bacon fat in the skillet and cook until the vegetables are very tender, about 5 minutes. Add ¼ cup of the chicken broth, the Worcestershire, and the remaining teaspoon of Tabasco. In a separate bowl, blend the cornstarch with the remaining ¼ cup broth; add to the vegetables in the skillet. Cook, stirring constantly until smooth and thick, about 2 minutes. Add the shrimp to the sauce and cook until they begin to curl and turn pink, about 2 minutes. Stir in the green onions and continue cooking until the shrimp are opaque throughout. Place a scoop of hot stone-ground grits in a deep bowl and cover with shrimp and sauce.

Note: The grits I order from the Nora Mill Granary are excellent (see Sources, page 252).

seared scallop salad with mustard dressing

WLS ½ portion: Calories 154, fat 9 gr, carbs 5 gr, protein 13.5 gr
Serves 4

I find that most people who have bariatric surgery crave green vegetables in the 2- to 4-month range post-op, and this salad is satisfying. Scallops are moist and tender as long as they are seared until they are just cooked through. The tender spinach leaves are low in carbohydrates. The dressing is tangy and smooth. You can substitute shrimp or chunks of mahimahi for the scallops.

6 cups baby spinach leaves, rinsed and dried
1 ripe Hass avocado, halved lengthwise and cut crosswise into
**   half-moon slices**
1½ pounds large sea scallops, tough tendons removed
1 tablespoon olive oil
Kosher salt and freshly ground black pepper
2 garlic cloves, minced
½ teaspoon sweet paprika

¼ cup sour cream

2 tablespoons light mayonnaise

1 tablespoon Dijon mustard

Juice of 1 lemon, about 2 tablespoons

Make a small bed of baby spinach leaves and arrange the avocado slices on 4 dinner plates.

Preheat a large nonstick skillet over high heat. In a large bowl, toss the scallops with the olive oil, salt, pepper, garlic, and paprika. Sear the scallops a total of 3 to 4 minutes, turning once, until they are just opaque in the center. Reserving any pan juices, place a portion of broiled scallops on each salad. In a small bowl, combine the reserved scallop juices with the sour cream, mayonnaise, mustard, lemon juice, and salt and pepper to taste. Drizzle the dressing over the salads and serve.

salmon bruschetta

WLS ½ portion: Calories 166, fat 10 gr, carbs 2 gr, protein 15 gr
Serves 4

This recipe takes a richly flavored bruschetta salad that would be delicious on a piece of garlic toast and features it to accentuate a piece of perfectly roasted salmon. For this dish, I love the taste of the giant Cerignola olives.

Four 5- to 6-ounce salmon fillets

Kosher salt and freshly ground black pepper

3 tablespoons olive oil

⅔ cup black olive pieces, Cerignola or Kalamata
   (see Note, page 113)

3 ripe Roma tomatoes, diced

½ small red onion, minced

1 tablespoon balsamic vinegar
1 tablespoon julienned basil
1 garlic clove, minced

Preheat the oven to 425°F. Arrange the fillets on a baking sheet, season with salt and pepper, and roast 8 to 10 minutes per 1 inch of thickness, until the fish is just opaque throughout.

Combine the olives, tomatoes, onion, olive oil, vinegar, basil, and garlic in a medium bowl. Place the roasted fillets in the center of each plate and heap with the bruschetta mixture.

salmon baked in salsa verde

WLS ½ portion: Calories 145, fat 7.5 gr, carbs 3 gr, protein 16 gr
Serves 4

This dish is commonplace in Mexico but is usually prepared with grouper or snapper. I love the color and flavor contrast using a piece of fresh wild salmon. The salsa verde keeps the fish extremely moist. I serve this beautiful dish accompanied with yellow rice and seasoned black beans.

Four 5- to 6-ounce salmon fillets
Kosher salt and freshly ground black pepper
2 garlic cloves
1 poblano chile, stemmed, seeded, and chopped
¾ cup chopped cilantro, lightly packed
¾ cup chopped flat-leaf parsley, lightly packed
6 green onions (scallions), sliced
1 tablespoon white vinegar
2 ripe Roma tomatoes, diced
½ teaspoon dried oregano
2 tablespoons olive oil

Preheat the oven to 425°F. Season the fish with salt and pepper and place in a shallow baking dish. Combine the garlic, chile, cilantro, parsley, green onions, vinegar, tomatoes, oregano, and olive oil in a blender or food processor and coarsely puree. Season with salt and pepper. Pour the salsa verde mixture over the fish and bake 25 to 30 minutes, until the fish is opaque throughout. Carefully remove the fillets to serving plates and spoon some of the sauce over the top.

roasted salmon
with tzatziki sauce

WLS ½ portion: Calories 144, fat 7 gr, carbs 3 gr, protein 16 gr
Serves 4

This cool cucumber–garlic sauce is one of my favorites. It is perfect for a beautifully roasted piece of salmon; the garlic, tart yogurt, and cucumber are a classic combination. If you have any of the tzatziki left over, serve it with pita bread wedges that you have baked to a golden crisp in a 350°F oven. I will roast an entire side of salmon fillet, and use the leftovers for a fast and delicious lunch entrée. Just flake the cold salmon, toss it with some of the tzatziki sauce, and serve it over a bed of baby spinach leaves that have been dressed with a little olive oil and lemon juice.

1 medium cucumber, peeled and seeded
½ cup low-fat yogurt
2 tablespoons light mayonnaise
Juice of ½ lemon, about 1 tablespoon
4 garlic cloves, mashed to a paste with a little salt

3 green onions (scallions), thinly sliced, including tender
   green tops
2 tablespoons chopped fresh dill
Kosher salt and freshly ground black pepper
Four 5- to 6-ounce salmon fillets

Preheat the oven to 425°F. Grate the cucumber using the large holes
on a box grater and squeeze to remove excess liquid. Place in a large
bowl and combine with the yogurt, mayonnaise, lemon juice, garlic,
green onions, and dill; add salt and plenty of black pepper. Arrange
the fish on a baking sheet and season with salt and pepper. Roast for 8
to 10 minutes, until just opaque throughout. Transfer the fish to serving plates and spoon some of the tzatziki sauce on top.

salmon burgers with artichoke tartar sauce

*WLS ½ portion: Calories 161, fat 10 gr, carbs 3 gr,
protein 16 gr
Serves 4*

This is a different but simple way to prepare heart-healthy
salmon. I buy wild salmon whenever it is available, but as long as
the farm raised is impeccably fresh it is reliable and delicious.
The artichoke tartar sauce is simply scrumptious; I use it as a
sauce for sautéed or grilled shrimp and scallops as a quick
supper.

burgers

1 ¼ to 1 ½ pounds salmon fillet, trimmed of skin, with pin bones
removed

2 tablespoons light mayonnaise

1 tablespoon chopped fresh dill

½ teaspoon kosher salt

½ teaspoon freshly ground black pepper

sauce

4 whole canned artichoke hearts, well drained and finely diced

¼ cup light mayonnaise

1 tablespoon minced red onion

1 tablespoon small capers, rinsed, drained, and coarsely chopped

1 teaspoon fresh lemon juice

1 tablespoon minced sweet pickle (Mt. Olive Pickle Company
makes a no-sugar-added sweet gherkin using Splenda)

1 tablespoon chopped flat-leaf parsley

Vegetable oil cooking spray

Coarsely grind the salmon in a food processor by pulsing on and off.
Transfer to a bowl, fold in the mayonnaise, dill, salt, and pepper, and
form into four ½-inch-thick patties. Cover and refrigerate for 1 hour to
make the burgers easier to handle.

Mix the artichokes, mayonnaise, onion, capers, lemon juice, pickle,
and parsley in a medium bowl until well combined; cover and chill
until serving.

Preheat a lightly oiled nonstick skillet over medium-high heat. Sear
the salmon burgers until the fish is just cooked throughout, 2 to 3 minutes per side. Place the burgers on plates and top with some of the sauce.

roasted salmon
with mango salsa

WLS ½ portion: Calories 153, fat 8 gr, carbs 6 gr, protein 15 gr
Serves 4

Mango salsa is my all-time favorite. I love to combine the
sweetness of fresh fruit with savory flavors and citrus as an
accompaniment for fish, seafood, and meats. Mango is very juicy
and makes the fish wonderfully moist. When the backyard mango
trees in my area are heavy with fruit, my friends bring me
shopping bags full in hopes of being rewarded with a big bowl of
this salsa. A tiny piece of grilled salmon with a spoonful of mango
salsa was one of my first soft food meals after my surgery. Roast a
double portion of the salmon and use the leftovers to make a
salmon–mango salad for the next day's lunch by flaking the cold
fillet and combining with a few spoonfuls of the salsa.

1 large ripe mango
Juice of 2 limes, 3 to 4 tablespoons
½ cup chopped fresh cilantro
1 small red onion, minced
2 tablespoons plus 1 teaspoon extra-virgin olive oil
Kosher salt and freshly ground black pepper
Several pinches of ground chipotle chile or cayenne, or a few
   dashes of Tabasco Chipotle sauce
Four 5- to 6-ounce salmon fillets

Preheat the oven to 425°F.

Peel the skin from the mango, slice off each fleshy half parallel to
the flat seed, and cut into even, ½-inch dice. Mix the diced mango

with the lime juice, cilantro, onion, and 2 tablespoons of the oil, adding salt, pepper, and hot pepper to taste.

Rub the salmon with the remaining teaspoon of olive oil, arrange on a baking sheet, and season with salt and pepper. Roast for 8 to 10 minutes per 1 inch of thickness of salmon fillet, measuring at the thickest point. Transfer to plates and spoon on the mango salsa.

grilled salmon
with wasabi sauce

WLS ½ portion: Calories 150, fat 8 gr, carbs 2 gr, protein 16 gr
Serves 4

I am a serious fan of wasabi, the pungent green Japanese horseradish. This quick sauce is sharp and creamy; a perfect companion for the soy–sesame glazed salmon fillet. Adjust the amount of wasabi to your taste. This sauce is also delicious as a dip for grilled skewered garlic shrimp or to drizzle over soy–sesame marinated chicken.

¾ cup soy sauce

1 tablespoon sesame oil

Four 5- to 6-ounce salmon fillets

1 tablespoon Japanese wasabi powder or 2 teaspoons
   prepared paste

¼ cup reduced fat sour cream

2 tablespoons light mayonnaise (see Note, page 112)

Kosher salt and freshly ground black pepper

3 green onions (scallions), thinly sliced

Blend the soy sauce with the sesame oil and pour over the salmon in a shallow dish. Marinate the salmon for 30 to 60 minutes.

In a small bowl, mix the wasabi powder with enough warm water to make a smooth, thick paste. Whisk in the sour cream and mayonnaise, then season with salt and pepper to taste. Add a little water to bring the mixture to a sauce consistency.

Preheat a grill pan or large nonstick skillet. Remove the fillets from the marinade and pat dry with paper towels. Place the fillets in the hot grill pan flesh-side down, and sear for 4 minutes. Carefully turn and cook the fillets for an additional 4 minutes, or until just barely cooked throughout. Transfer to plates, drizzle with wasabi sauce, and sprinkle with the sliced scallions.

catfish with
spicy orange sauce

WLS ½ portion: Calories 140, fat 9 gr, carbs 4 gr, protein 11 gr
Serves 4

Catfish is a meaty, mild fish, always available. This recipe pairs essential Asian flavors with orange juice, and can be put together in minutes while you dress some baby greens in the sesame dressing from page 180.

½ cup orange juice

1 tablespoon hoisin sauce, a sweet spicy Asian barbeque-style sauce, available in most supermarkets

2 tablespoons soy sauce

¼ cup sherry or Chinese cooking wine

1 teaspoon grated fresh ginger

1 garlic clove, minced

4 green onions (scallions), thinly sliced

2 teaspoons peanut oil

Four 5- to 6-ounce catfish fillets

All-purpose or Wondra flour for dusting

In a small bowl, blend the orange juice, hoisin sauce, soy sauce, and sherry; then stir in the ginger, garlic, and green onions. Heat the peanut oil over high heat in a large nonstick covered skillet or wok. Dry the fillets with paper towels and lightly dust with flour, patting off excess. Sear for 2 minutes, turn the fillets, and sear for 2 minutes more. Reduce the heat; add the sauce and simmer, covered, for 6 to 8 minutes, until the fish is opaque throughout. Transfer the fish to plates and spoon the sauce over.

roasted tilapia
with green chile crema

WLS ½ portion: Calories 97, fat 4 gr, carbs 2 gr, protein 18 gr
Serves 4

This simple sour cream-based sauce uses canned roasted green chiles and is delicious with a tilapia fillet. The sauce can be combined in minutes while the fish cooks, making this a perfect midweek meal. For your family, serve with yellow rice and seasoned black beans with garlic in olive oil.

Four 5- to 6-ounce tilapia fillets

1 teaspoon olive oil

Kosher salt and freshly ground black pepper

One 4-ounce can roasted mild green chiles, well drained, or
  ½ cup roasted salsa verde (see Note, page 107)

½ cup reduced-fat sour cream
¼ cup chopped cilantro
Juice of 1 lime, 1½ to 2 tablespoons

Preheat the oven to 425°F. Rub the fillets with olive oil, and season with salt and pepper. Roast for 6 to 8 minutes, until opaque through-out. Pulse the chiles, sour cream, cilantro, and lime juice in a food pro-cessor, and season to taste with salt and pepper. Transfer the fish to plates and spoon on the green chile crema.

simple flounder with salsa

WLS ½ portion: Calories 86, fat 3 gr, carbs 2 gr, protein 13 gr
Serves 4

My easiest recipe! This one can be on the table in barely 5 minutes. Flounder fillets are very thin and can be sautéed in just a minute or two. Choose fillets that are 5 to 6 ounces each so you won't have to sauté more than one per person.

The taste of this finished dish varies with the kind of salsa you use. Try roasted garlic, fire-roasted tomato, tomatillo, or chipotle varieties. I am always on the lookout for unusual small-batch salsas to have on hand when I need to prepare a quick meal. Make sure you read the salsa label and avoid those with black beans, peaches, corn, and sweeteners, or you will unnecessarily increase your carbohydrate count. This simple preparation also works with shrimp, scallops, or any sautéed fillet.

Four 5- to 6-ounce flounder fillets; if fillets are smaller, serve 2
**   per person**
Kosher salt and freshly ground black pepper
All-purpose or Wondra flour for dusting
1 tablespoon olive oil

1 garlic clove, slivered

1 cup prepared salsa (see Note, page 107)

Juice of one lime, 1½ to 2 tablespoons

1 tablespoon chopped cilantro or flat-leaf parsley

Season the fillets with salt and pepper; lightly dust with flour and pat off any excess. Heat the oil in a nonstick skillet over medium-high heat; sauté the fillets for 2 minutes, carefully turn, cook an additional minute or until just opaque throughout, and transfer to plates. Add the garlic to the skillet; sauté 1 minute, or until lightly browned. Add the salsa, lime juice, and cilantro to the skillet and cook until bubbling and hot. Pour the sauce over the fish fillets, and serve immediately.

roasted grouper with tomatoes and herbed cream sauce

WLS ½ portion: Calories 134, fat 6.6 gr, carbs 6 gr, protein 16 gr
Serves 4

Grouper is usually available where I live in Florida, but feel free to substitute tilapia, snapper, or salmon if it is the better choice in your area. This is a very attractive dish with a colorful contrast between the cream sauce and the marinated tomato topping and would be an excellent meal for company served with couscous and sautéed zucchini slices.

2 large shallots, minced

Juice of 2 lemons, about ¼ cup

1 tablespoon white wine vinegar

1 cup evaporated low-fat milk

2 teaspoons minced fresh thyme

Kosher salt and freshly ground black pepper

2 ripe Roma tomatoes, finely diced

2 tablespoons olive oil

1 tablespoon julienned fresh basil

Four 5- to 6-ounce grouper fillets

Combine half of the shallots, 2 tablespoons of the lemon juice, and the vinegar in small saucepan. Boil over medium-high heat until the liquid is reduced to a glaze, about 4 minutes. Add the the milk and thyme, bring the mixture to a boil, reduce the heat, and simmer for 4 to 5 minutes, until thickened to a sauce consistency. Season with salt and pepper and set aside.

Combine the tomatoes, oil, and basil with the remaining shallots and lemon juice in a small bowl. Season with salt and pepper and set aside.

Preheat the oven to 425°F. Season the fish with salt and pepper and arrange on a baking sheet. Roast for 8 to 10 minutes per inch of thickness, until the fish is opaque throughout. Transfer the fillets to serving plates. Spoon the warm cream sauce around the fish and mound some of the tomato mixture on top of each fillet.

grouper with red pepper coulis

WLS ½ portion: Calories 76, fat <1 gr, carbs 3 gr, protein 14 gr
Serves 4

This sauce has a wonderful Asian flavor that accents the
sweetness of the red pepper and highlights a simply prepared
piece of fish. Grouper is delicious, but buy whatever is freshest at
your fish market; swordfish, salmon, flounder, shrimp, or scallops
would be perfect when simply seasoned, grilled, and placed in a
pool of this snappy red sauce. This meal can be completed with
jasmine or basmati rice and snow peas that are quickly stir-fried
in a teaspoon of peanut oil with garlic slivers.

2 red bell peppers, quartered, stems and seeds removed
½ medium onion, sliced
1 tablespoon grated fresh ginger
1 teaspoon Tabasco sauce
1 tablespoon rice wine vinegar
Kosher salt and pepper to taste
Vegetable oil cooking spray
Four 5- to 6-ounce grouper fillets

Combine the peppers, onion, and ginger with ¾ cup water in a
medium saucepan and bring to a boil. Reduce the heat, cover, and simmer until the peppers are very soft, about 12 minutes. Remove the
peppers and onion with a slotted spoon and puree in food processor.
Blend in the Tabasco and vinegar, and season with salt and pepper.

Preheat the broiler or a lightly sprayed nonstick grill pan. Broil the
grouper no more than 8 to 10 minutes per inch of thickness, or grill in
a grill pan, until just opaque throughout. Spoon a puddle of pepper
puree on each plate and center a fish fillet on top of the sauce.

mahimahi with puttanesca sauce

WLS ½ portion: Calories 100, fat 3 gr, carbs 5 gr, protein 14 gr
Serves 4

This is a wonderful sauce for any firm meaty type fish, including grouper and swordfish. Do not shy away from this classic sauce because of the anchovies—they melt into the sauce and add a mellow saltiness that cannot be duplicated. Serve with a mixed tossed salad dressed with balsamic vinegar and olive oil.

1 tablespoon olive oil
2 garlic cloves, minced
1 medium red onion, thinly sliced
4 anchovy fillets, rinsed and minced
One 14-ounce can diced tomatoes, drained
⅓ cup oil-cured black Kalamata olive pieces (see Note, page 113)
2 tablespoons small capers, rinsed
1 teaspoon finely chopped fresh rosemary
Kosher salt and freshly ground black pepper
Four 5- to 6-ounce mahimahi pieces, cut 1 inch thick, with skin removed
⅓ cup chopped flat-leaf parsley
Pinch of crushed red pepper

Preheat the oven to 425°F. Heat the olive oil in a medium saucepan over medium-high heat and sauté the garlic and onion until softened, about 4 minutes. Add the anchovies and cook until they have softened to a paste, about 2 minutes. Stir in the tomatoes, olives, capers, and rosemary. Bring the sauce to a boil, reduce the heat, and simmer 5 minutes. Add salt and pepper to taste.

Arrange the fish pieces on a baking sheet and season with salt and pepper. Roast the fish for 8 to 10 minutes, until just cooked throughout. Place a piece of fish in the center of each plate. Stir the parsley and crushed red pepper into the sauce and spoon over the fish.

swordfish with charred tomato vinaigrette

WLS ½ portion: Calories 181, fat 10 gr, carbs 3 gr, protein 18 gr
Serves 4

Swordfish is my favorite fish. My local fish market sells its swordfish steaks trimmed into 4- to 6-ounce serving pieces with the tough skin and darker center flesh removed, which makes the preparation even easier. The tomato vinaigrette from this recipe is perfect with any broiled or grilled fish or shellfish; the roasted tomato flavor is fantastic when paired with skewers of grilled shrimp. Or use it on roasted and thinly sliced turkey breast.

4 large ripe Roma tomatoes, cut in half lengthwise
1 small red onion, sliced
3 garlic cloves, left whole
1 teaspoon chopped fresh basil
1 teaspoon chopped fresh thyme
1½ tablespoons balsamic vinegar
¼ cup extra-virgin olive oil
Kosher salt and freshly ground black pepper
Four 5- to 6-ounce swordfish pieces, cut 1 inch thick, trimmed
　　with skin removed

Preheat the broiler. Arrange the tomatoes cut side down along with the onion slices and garlic on a baking sheet. Broil 12 to 15 minutes, until the tops of the vegetables are charred and juices are released. Remove from the broiler and pour the contents of the pan, including juices, into a food processor; add the basil and thyme and pulse until the sauce is blended but still has some texture. Transfer the mixture to a bowl, stir in the vinegar and olive oil, and add salt and pepper to taste.

Season the fish with salt and pepper and broil for 8 to 10 minutes until the fish is opaque throughout. Transfer the fish pieces to plates and spoon the charred tomato vinaigrette over the swordfish.

swordfish steaks with cilantro cream

WLS ½ portion: Calories 145, fat 5.5 gr, carbs 3 gr, protein 20 gr
Serves 4

The cilantro cream is the star of this meal, making a piece of impeccably fresh grilled fish into something extraordinary. I wouldn't hesitate to substitute grouper, flounder, jumbo shrimp, or sea scallops. For the others in your family, serve with saffron rice and ripe tomato slices.

1 teaspoon olive oil
2 large shallots, sliced
4 garlic cloves, sliced
⅔ cup chopped cilantro, lightly packed
½ cup low-sodium chicken broth
½ cup evaporated low-fat milk
Kosher salt and freshly ground black pepper
Four 5- to 6-ounce swordfish pieces, cut about 1 inch thick, trimmed of skin

Heat the olive oil in a small saucepan over medium-high heat and sauté the shallots and garlic until softened. Add the cilantro and toss for 15 seconds. Stir in the broth and milk, and cook for 1 minute to steep the herbs. Transfer the mixture to a blender, and tightly holding the lid with a kitchen towel, blend until the sauce is smooth. Return the sauce to the pan, bring to a boil, reduce the heat, and simmer, stirring occasionally, until it begins to thicken. Season to taste with salt and pepper, and set aside. Preheat the broiler or a grill pan. Cook the swordfish 5 to 6 minutes per side, until cooked throughout. Spoon some of the sauce on each plate and place a swordfish piece in the center.

Swordfish with Tarragon Cream
Substitute ⅓ cup fresh tarragon leaves for the cilantro and use a squeeze of fresh orange juice to season the fish.

halibut with
ginger–tahini sauce

WLS ½ portion: Calories 134.5, fat 7 gr, carbs 2 gr, protein 15 gr
Serves 4

I keep a jar of sesame paste—tahini—in my refrigerator to use for hummus, and wanted to find another use for this toasty nut butter. This vinaigrette combines the distinctive Asian flavors of sesame, pickled ginger, soy sauce, and green onion. For your family, pair this with steamed rice and some roasted asparagus spears. I can find jars of pickled ginger in my local supermarket; however, the ginger at my local sushi bar tastes much better. When we go for sushi, I ask the chef for a small plastic to-go cup and he is always happy to oblige. You can substitute salmon or swordfish.

1 teaspoon whole cumin seeds

2 tablespoons peanut oil

1 garlic clove, minced

2 tablespoons tahini (sesame paste)

1 tablespoon soy sauce

Juice of 2 limes, 3 to 4 tablespoons

2 green onions (scallions), thinly sliced

¼ cup finely chopped pickled ginger, also called *gari*

Kosher salt and freshly ground black pepper

**Four 5- to 6-ounce halibut pieces, cut 1 inch thick, trimmed with
    skin removed**

Toast the cumin seeds in a dry skillet over medium-high heat, moving the pan constantly, until it is fragrant. Transfer the cumin seeds to a bowl. In a large bowl, whisk together the cumin, peanut oil, garlic, tahini, soy sauce, lime juice, and 3 tablespoons water, then stir in the green onions and ginger. Season with salt and pepper. Marinate the fish for 30 to 45 minutes in ¼ cup of the marinade.

Preheat the oven to 425°F. Shake the marinade from the fish pieces. Arrange the fish on a baking sheet and roast 8 to 10 minutes, until cooked through but still moist. Serve the fish with a little of the remaining ginger–tahini mixture as a sauce.

spiced tuna steaks with fennel and red pepper sauté

WLS ½ portion: Calories 113, fat 3 gr, carbs 4 gr, protein 18 gr
Serves 4

A seared, meaty tuna steak with a fennel-and-black pepper crust
is accompanied by a sautéed fennel and sweet red pepper
condiment. Do not overcook the tuna; just a minute of additional

heat can turn a delectable moist ruby-colored tuna fillet into a dry brown hockey puck.

Four 5- to 6-ounce tuna steaks, cut 1 inch thick
1 tablespoon plus 1 teaspoon olive oil, plus extra for coating the tuna
1 tablespoon whole fennel seeds
1½ teaspoons whole black peppercorns
1 medium fennel bulb, trimmed, cut into quarters, cored, and
   thinly sliced lengthwise
1 medium red bell pepper, cut into quarters and thinly sliced
2 garlic cloves, sliced
1 tablespoon fresh lemon juice (about ½ lemon)
Kosher salt and freshly ground black pepper

Lightly rub one side of each piece of tuna with the oil. Crush the fennel seeds and peppercorns with the bottom of a small heavy skillet on a cutting board; press some of the coarse mixture onto the oiled side of each tuna steak and set aside. Heat 1 tablespoon of the olive oil in a covered skillet over medium-high heat. Sauté the fennel, red pepper, and garlic, stirring occasionally, until lightly browned, about 4 minutes. Add ¼ cup water, cover, reduce the heat, and simmer the vegetables 10 minutes, until the fennel is very tender. Uncover and boil until the liquid is nearly evaporated. Stir in the lemon juice, season with salt and pepper, and remove from the heat.

Heat a teaspoon of olive oil in a large nonstick skillet over high heat just until it begins to smoke. Add the tuna steaks spice side down, and sear, undisturbed, for 30 seconds; reduce the heat to medium-high and continue to cook for 1½ minutes. Carefully turn and sear the second side for an additional 1½ minutes. Remove the tuna steaks to a cutting board, and immediately cut each piece across the grain into ½-inch-thick slices. The tuna should be rare to medium-rare in the center. Fan the tuna pieces on each plate and spoon some of the fennel–pepper mixture to the side.

chicken and turkey

Chicken and turkey are excellent sources of protein. One boneless, skinless chicken thigh weighs approximately 2½ ounces and provides approximately 18 grams of lean protein. Of course, breast meat has fewer grams of fat, but it is drier in texture and is therefore more difficult to eat during those first post-op months. Turkey is even a little higher in protein content with 2½ ounces containing more than 20 grams of protein. Cornish game hens are super-moist when marinated, have very tender meat, and can be substituted for the chicken and turkey in several of the roasted recipes.

With all the problems people say they have with eating chicken in their early post-surgery months, you might wonder why a chapter on poultry is included. Having trouble eating certain foods is largely due to the texture of a dish and this, of course, has a great deal to do with how the food is cooked. When I ask my weight loss surgery friends how the offending chicken was prepared, it was usually white meat, baked, broiled, or fried, and served plain. Aha! Chicken thighs are very moist and much easier to digest than breasts, so many of the recipes here use either boneless or whole thighs. I almost always use chicken thighs at home as my first choice, and only started cooking breasts again eighteen months post-op. I occasionally have a tough time eating chicken breasts; I have tried brining them, marinating them, poaching them, and saucing them, but they are just too dense in consistency—I can only eat a few bites before I have an uncomfortable feeling of fullness and indigestion.

Consider the consistency of a bite of oven-baked chicken breast; then think about the texture of chicken cacciatore, the chicken thighs simmered in tomato sauce until tender. Which would you choose?

An instant-read thermometer is inexpensive, and indispensable. You will marvel at how juicy a boneless roasted turkey breast really is when it is perfectly cooked to an internal temperature of 160°F. Roast a whole chicken, turkey, or game hen until the thickest part of the thigh is cooked to an internal temperature of 170°F. I now buy organic chicken parts; I can buy exactly the amount I like. I also prefer that the chickens are fed an organic diet with no antibiotics. They are tastier than the supermarket chicken, and with the small portions we eat post-op, quality is important.

These recipes serve four people who have not had gastric bypass surgery. The person who is eating after having had bypass surgery would be eating about one half of one serving. For example, a recipe using 8 large chicken thighs would feed 4 people, serving two thighs per person; the WLS ½ portion would be one thigh with enough of the sauce to moisten it. The nutritional analysis has been calculated for the WLS ½ portion including the sauce for that dish.

chicken cutlets with sun-dried tomato dijon sauce

WLS ½ portion: Calories 119, fat 6 gr, carbs 3 gr, protein 15.5 gr
Serves 4

Pounding the chicken cutlets tenderizes them. I buy whole boneless breasts, which I split horizontally with a sharp knife to butterfly, and then pound between sheets of plastic wrap or wax

paper. If you don't have a meat mallet, use a small, heavy pot or a
rolling pin. I serve this to family with a side dish of spinach
sautéed with garlic in olive oil, and Yukon gold mashed potatoes.

4 boneless, skinless chicken breast halves, about 1½ pounds
Kosher salt and freshly ground black pepper
All-purpose or Wondra flour for dusting
2 tablespoons olive oil
2 garlic cloves, thinly sliced
¼ cup finely diced sun-dried tomatoes, about 6 pieces
2 tablespoons Dijon mustard
½ cup evaporated low-fat milk
½ cup low-sodium chicken broth

Butterfly the chicken breast halves, and then pound to an even ½-inch
thickness. Season the chicken with salt and pepper and dust very
lightly with flour. Heat the olive oil in a large nonstick skillet over
medium-high heat and sauté the chicken cutlets until browned on
both sides and cooked through, about 2 minutes per side. Transfer
them to a serving platter.

In the oil remaining in the skillet, sauté the garlic until softened,
about 2 minutes. Reduce the heat to low, add the sun-dried tomatoes
and mustard; whisk in the evaporated milk and broth. Heat gently
until the sauce thickens, stirring constantly, adding the accumulated
juices from the chicken platter. Do not boil the sauce or it will separate.

Return the chicken cutlets to the pan and turn to coat with the
sauce. Season with salt and pepper and serve immediately.

roasted chicken chipotle salad

WLS ½ portion: Calories 147, fat 3 gr, carbs <1 gr, protein 14 gr
Serves 4

A perfect salad for a lunch with my girlfriends! I started eating salad early after my surgery—the leaves are tender and the dressing makes it very moist. Eat the chicken first, and when you start getting full, nibble on a few shreds of lettuce and pieces of avocado. The blue corn tortilla crisps add just enough crunch along with a beautiful color contrast, but if you cannot find the blue tortillas, substitute white or yellow. I arrange this salad in a large bowl, then add the dressing at the last minute and toss to coat at the table; I divide the salad among individual plates and top each with a few of the blue corn tortilla shreds.

4 large chicken breast halves, about 2 pounds
Kosher salt and freshly ground black pepper
½ teaspoon chili powder (I use pure ground chipotle)
¼ cup light or reduced-fat mayonnaise
Juice of 1 lime, 1½ to 2 tablespoons
3 canned chipotle chiles in adobo sauce, scraped of seeds and
   finely minced
1 garlic clove, minced
2 tablespoons chopped cilantro
Chicken broth, optional
1 large head romaine lettuce, torn into small pieces or
   shredded
1 ripe Hass avocado, peeled and cut into 1-inch cubes
½ cup grape tomatoes, cut in half
2 blue corn tortillas, cut into ¼-inch strips, salted and baked at
   350°F until crisp

Preheat the oven to 400°F. Loosen the skin from the chicken but do not remove. Season the meat with salt, pepper, and chili powder, place on a baking sheet, and roast for 35 to 40 minutes, until the juices run clear when pierced with the tip of a knife or an instant-read thermometer registers 160°F. Set aside. When the chicken is cool enough to handle, remove the skin and bones and pull the meat apart into large pieces. Puree the mayonnaise, lime juice, chipotles, garlic, and cilantro in a blender or food processor, adding a little water or chicken broth for a slightly thinner consistency. Season with salt and pepper.

Arrange the lettuce, avocado, and tomatoes on plates; add some of the shredded chicken, drizzle with the chipotle dressing, and pile on a few crisp tortilla pieces.

jerk chicken with black bean and red pepper sauté

WLS ½ portion: Calories 151, fat 6 gr, carbs 9 gr, protein 16 gr
Serves 4

We have traveled to the islands of the Caribbean throughout the years, which has given me the chance to sample jerk marinades in numerous locations. I love the contrasts of the citrus, herbs, and spices in this Jamaican dish. This dish requires advance preparation.

4 large chicken breast halves, about 2 pounds
4 green onions (scallions), thinly sliced
3 garlic cloves, crushed
3 jalapeño chiles, stemmed, seeded, and minced
Juice of 2 limes, 3 to 4 tablespoons
Juice of 1 orange, about ⅓ cup
2 tablespoons chopped fresh thyme or 2 teaspoons dried thyme

3 tablespoons olive oil

¼ teaspoon freshly ground black pepper, plus additional to taste

½ teaspoon cayenne

½ teaspoon ground cinnamon

¼ teaspoon ground allspice

1 red bell pepper, diced

1 small red onion, diced

One 15-ounce can black beans, rinsed and drained

½ cup low-sodium chicken broth

Kosher salt

Loosen the skin on the chicken breasts but do not remove. Place the green onions, 2 of the garlic cloves, 2 of the jalapeños, the juice of 1 lime (1½ to 2 tablespoons), orange juice, thyme, 2 tablespoons of the olive oil, pepper, cayenne, cinnamon, and allspice in a food processor and pulse to combine. Pour the jerk marinade over the chicken in a deep bowl or plastic bag, and refrigerate for 4 to 24 hours.

Preheat the oven to 425°F. Drain the chicken; arrange the pieces on a baking sheet and roast for 30 to 35 minutes, until the juices run clear when pierced with the tip of a knife or an instant-read thermometer registers 160°F.

Heat the remaining 1 tablespoon olive oil in a medium skillet over medium-high heat and sauté the remaining jalapeño and garlic clove, along with the red pepper and onion until lightly browned and softened, about 5 minutes. Stir in the beans, the remaining lime juice, and the chicken broth, slightly mashing the vegetables together. Reduce the heat and simmer for 15 minutes. Season with salt and pepper.

When the chicken is cool enough to handle, remove the skin and bones and cut into thick slices. To serve, spoon some of the black bean and red pepper sauté on a plate and arrange the chicken slices on top.

chicken marsala

WLS ½ portion: Calories 114, fat 4 gr, carbs 2 gr, protein 15 gr
Serves 4

Serve this to family over a pile of thin spaghetti dressed with a
little olive oil, salt, pepper, red pepper flakes, and parsley;
steamed broccoli adds low-carbohydrate nutrition and color.

4 boneless, skinless chicken breast halves, about 1½ pounds
Kosher salt and freshly ground black pepper
All-purpose or Wondra flour for dusting
1 tablespoon olive oil
1 tablespoon salted butter
1 small onion, finely diced
8 ounces crimini or button mushrooms, sliced
½ cup Marsala wine
½ cup low-sodium chicken broth
1 teaspoon cornstarch dissolved in 1 tablespoon water
2 tablespoons chopped flat-leaf parsley

Butterfly the chicken breast halves, and pound to an even ½-inch
thickness. Season the chicken with salt and pepper and dust lightly
with flour. Heat the olive oil in a large nonstick skillet over medium-
high heat and sauté the chicken cutlets until lightly browned on both
sides, about 2 minutes per side; transfer to a serving platter when finished. Add the butter to the remaining olive oil in the same pan, and
sauté the onion and mushrooms until the liquid has evaporated and
the mushrooms start to brown, about 4 minutes. Add the wine, chicken
broth, and the chicken with any accumulated juices from the platter,
and simmer 3 to 4 minutes, until the chicken is cooked through.
Transfer the chicken back to the serving platter; thicken the sauce with

the cornstarch mixture. Stir in the parsley and pour the sauce over the chicken.

chicken with
dijon–orange sauce

WLS ½ portion: Calories 91, fat 3 gr, carbs 2.5 gr, protein 14 gr
Serves 4

Tender chicken cutlets with a sweet and sharp sauce can be quickly prepared and on the table in just 15 minutes. It pairs perfectly with a simple tossed salad with balsamic vinaigrette and spinach sautéed in olive oil with garlic.

4 boneless, skinless chicken breast halves, about 1½ pounds
Kosher salt and freshly ground black pepper
All-purpose or Wondra flour for dusting
1 tablespoon olive oil
1 garlic clove, minced
½ cup orange juice
2 tablespoons Dijon mustard
2 tablespoons Smucker's Light Sugar Free Apricot Preserves
½ teaspoon Tabasco sauce
2 green onions (scallions), thinly sliced

Butterfly the chicken breast halves, and pound to an even ½-inch thickness. Season the chicken with salt and pepper and dust lightly with flour. Heat the olive oil in a large nonstick skillet over medium-high heat and sauté the chicken cutlets until lightly browned on both sides and cooked through, about 2 minutes per side; transfer to a serving platter. Sauté the garlic in the oil remaining in the pan for 1 minute; stir

in the orange juice, mustard, preserves, Tabasco, and green onions.
Bring to a boil and cook until the sauce has thickened, about 4 minutes. Return the chicken to the skillet, coat with sauce, and simmer
until heated through.

pollo acapulco, chicken simmered in ancho–guajillo sauce

WLS ½ portion: Calories 127, fat 5 gr, carbs 6 gr, protein 14.5 gr
Serves 4

This recipe was inspired by several large bags of dried chiles, in
shades of red from vermilion to mahogany, brought home from a
Mexican vacation. It is delicious with various combinations of
dried peppers, but try to use some of the sweeter varieties; this
dish is about flavor, not heat. I have made the dish with only
ancho chiles and have even added a few dried chipotles for
different but equally delicious results. The texture of the
simmered chicken is very easy for people to eat early after
bariatric surgery and is a perfect meal for my family served with
herbed rice and a salad.

3 dried ancho chiles (See Sources, page 250)
3 dried guajillo chiles (See Sources, page 250)
2 tablespoons olive oil
1 large sweet onion, chopped
5 cloves garlic, sliced
One 14-ounce can diced tomatoes, drained (see Note,
  page 122)

8 large bone-in, skinless chicken thighs, about 2 pounds
Kosher salt and freshly ground black pepper
½ cup chopped cilantro

Tear the dried chiles into large flat pieces, removing and discarding the stems and seeds. Toast the chile pieces a few seconds, one at a time, in a nonstick skillet over medium-high heat, pressing down with a spatula until slight wisps of smoke appear. Transfer the toasted chiles to a small deep bowl, cover with 1 cup of very hot water to soften, and set aside while preparing the remaining ingredients.

Heat 1 tablespoon of the olive oil in a covered skillet over medium-high heat and sauté the onion and garlic until lightly browned and softened, about 5 minutes. Add the tomatoes, bring to a boil, reduce the heat, and simmer 5 minutes. Place the drained chiles and the tomato-onion mixture in a blender, and puree until very smooth. Set aside. (Be careful when blending hot liquids: always tightly hold down the lid with a kitchen towel, because the hot liquids will expand when blended; it is safest to pulse the mixture.)

Season the chicken pieces with salt and pepper and brown in a nonstick covered skillet with the remaining tablespoon of olive oil over medium-high heat; drain any accumulated fat. Add the pureed sauce, cover the skillet, lower the heat, and simmer 45 minutes, or until the chicken is very tender. Transfer the chicken pieces to a platter. Stir the cilantro into the sauce, season with salt and pepper, and pour over the chicken.

Ancho-Guajillo Shrimp

This recipe makes enough sauce so that I can keep a generous cup aside and save it for a shrimp meal later in the week. I sauté a little chopped garlic in some olive oil, then add the reserved ancho-guajillo sauce and simmer for 20 minutes to smooth out the flavors; add 1¼ pounds of peeled and deveined shrimp and cook until the shrimp are just opaque, adding a handful of chopped cilantro just before serving.

baja roasted chicken
with spicy avocado crema

WLS ½ portion: Calories 131, fat 7 gr, carbs 3 gr, protein 14.5 gr
Serves 4

I love to use spice rubs on roasted meats. I serve this entrée with
saffron rice and a simple cherry tomato salad dressed with lime
juice and olive oil. Any extra Spicy Avocado Crema can be
enjoyed with tortilla chips.

1 tablespoon chopped cilantro
1 teaspoon poultry seasoning
1 teaspoon garlic powder
½ teaspoon sweet paprika
½ teaspoon kosher salt
½ teaspoon coarsely ground black pepper
¼ teaspoon crushed red pepper
1 tablespoon olive oil
8 large boneless, skinless chicken thighs, about
   1½ pounds

spicy avocado crema

1 large ripe Hass avocado, peeled and cut into
   chunks
2 garlic cloves, sliced
2 green onions (scallions), sliced
2 tablespoons chopped cilantro
¼ cup reduced-fat sour cream
Juice of 1 lime, 1½ to 2 tablespoons

Few dashes of Tabasco sauce
About ¼ cup low-sodium chicken broth
Kosher salt and freshly ground black pepper

Preheat the oven to 400°F. Combine the cilantro, poultry seasoning, garlic powder, paprika, salt, black pepper, red pepper, and olive oil in a small bowl, blending to form a paste. Rub a little of the mixture on each chicken thigh and arrange the thighs in a medium roasting pan. Roast without turning for 35 minutes, or until the chicken is golden brown and fork-tender.

Puree the avocado, garlic, green onions, and cilantro in a food processor. Add the sour cream, lime juice, Tabasco, and enough chicken broth to thin to a sauce consistency. Season with salt and pepper; add more Tabasco if desired. Thinly slice the chicken, arrange on plates, and drizzle with the Spicy Avocado Crema.

Spiced Roast Turkey Breast
The rub from this recipe is also delicious on a boneless roasted turkey breast. Have the butcher cut the meat from the frame of a 2½ to 3-pound turkey breast half for you if you don't want to do it yourself, although it is very simple. Make the spice paste and spread it on the turkey, then roll and tie with cotton string in several places to form an evenly shaped roast. Roast 45 to 60 minutes at 400°F, until the juices run clear or a thermometer reads an internal temperature of 160°F. Slice the roast, arrange on a platter and serve with the Spicy Avocado Crema as a sauce.

chicken tagine

WLS ½ portion: Calories 164, fat 6.5 gr, carbs 5 gr, protein 16 gr
Serves 4

The turmeric, paprika, and saffron tint the sauce a deep, golden orange, and the scent of the cumin, ginger, and cinnamon is rich and sweet in this Moroccan dish. When I serve this dish to my friends or family, I place a large scoop of couscous in a flat pasta bowl, topped by chicken, and then ladle on the chunky sauce. Round out the meal with a simple salad with lemon-olive oil vinaigrette.

8 large boneless, skinless chicken thighs, about 1½ pounds, cut into 2-inch pieces

Kosher salt and freshly ground black pepper

1 tablespoon olive oil

1 large onion, diced

4 garlic cloves, chopped

1 teaspoon ground ginger

1 teaspoon cumin

2 teaspoons sweet paprika

1 teaspoon ground turmeric

1 teaspoon ground cinnamon

1 cup low-sodium chicken broth

½ teaspoon saffron threads

Juice of 2 lemons, about ¼ cup

1 teaspoon cornstarch dissolved in 1 tablespoon water

1 tablespoon lemon zest

½ cup green olive pieces, freshly cut from the pit (see Note, page 113)

¼ cup blanched whole almonds

½ cup coarsely chopped flat-leaf parsley

Season the chicken with salt and pepper. Heat the olive oil in a Dutch oven or large covered nonstick skillet over medium-high heat. Brown the chicken pieces and remove to a plate. Pour off all but 1 tablespoon of the fat and sauté the onion and garlic until translucent, about 4 minutes. Stir in the ginger, cumin, paprika, turmeric, and cinnamon; cook for 1 minute, stirring constantly, and return the chicken to the pot with any accumulated juices. Stir in the broth, saffron, lemon juice, and ½ teaspoon salt; bring to a boil, cover, reduce the heat, and simmer for 35 to

40 minutes, until the chicken is very tender. Stir in the cornstarch mixture to thicken the sauce. Add the lemon zest, olives, almonds, and parsley; simmer an additional 5 minutes, check the seasonings, and serve.

garlic roasted chicken
with black olive tapenade

WLS ½ portion: Calories 151, fat 10 gr, carbs 1.5 gr, protein 14 gr
Serves 4

Black olives add a lot of flavor without high carbohydrates. This olive paste is rich and mellow with a lemon-and-garlic kick. Spread leftovers on flatbread crackers. Serve this dish with spinach sautéed in olive oil with garlic, and sliced ripe tomatoes.

3 garlic cloves
Kosher salt
3 tablespoons olive oil
Juice of ½ lemon, about 1 tablespoon
Freshly ground black pepper
8 large boneless, skinless chicken thighs, about 1½ pounds
¾ cup Niçoise olives, pitted (see Note, page 113)
2 anchovy fillets, rinsed
1 tablespoon pine nuts

Preheat the oven to 425°F. Mash 2 garlic cloves with a little salt on a cutting board with the side of a large chef's knife to create a paste. Transfer the garlic paste to a small bowl and blend with 1 tablespoon of the olive oil, 1 teaspoon of the lemon juice, and a few grinds of black pepper. Toss the chicken thighs with the garlic-oil mixture, arrange in a shallow roasting pan, and bake for 30 to 35 minutes, or until the juices run clear. Combine the remaining garlic clove, the remaining 2 teaspoons lemon juice, olives, anchovy fillets, and pine nuts in a food processor and pulse until a slightly textured paste forms. Transfer to a small bowl, stir in the remaining 2 tablespoons olive oil, and season with salt and pepper.

Thinly slice the chicken thighs, fan out on each plate, and serve with a few spoonfuls of the black olive tapenade to the side.

milanese chicken sauté

WLS ½ portion: Calories 132, fat 5 gr, carbs 6 gr, protein 14 gr
Serves 4

The inspiration for this recipe was a platter of meltingly tender osso buco, the Milanese veal dish I enjoyed at a New Jersey trattoria just before having my bariatric surgery. The braised shanks had great depth of flavor, but what got me was the sprinkling of gremolata, a mixture of finely chopped garlic, lemon zest, and parsley, that made this simple comfort food memorable.

8 large boneless, skinless chicken thighs, about 1½ pounds, cut into 2-inch pieces
Kosher salt and freshly ground black pepper
1 tablespoon olive oil
1 large onion, chopped
3 garlic cloves, chopped
1 medium carrot, quartered lengthwise and thinly sliced
½ cup white wine
One 14-ounce can diced tomatoes in juice
1 teaspoon dried thyme

1 bay leaf

Zest of 1 orange, cut with a vegetable peeler, scraped of white pith, and finely julienned

1 teaspoon cornstarch dissolved in 1 tablespoon water

gremolata

Finely grated zest of 1 lemon

3 tablespoons chopped flat-leaf parsley

1 garlic clove, very finely minced with a pinch of salt

Season the chicken with salt and pepper. Heat the olive oil in a Dutch oven or large covered nonstick skillet over medium-high heat. Brown the chicken pieces and transfer them to a bowl. Discard all but 1 tablespoon of fat from the pot; add the onion, garlic, and carrot, and cook until softened, about 4 minutes. Add the wine, tomatoes, thyme, bay leaf, orange zest, and the chicken, along with any accumulated juices. Bring to a boil, cover, reduce the heat, and simmer for 35 to 40 minutes until the chicken is very tender. Stir in the cornstarch mixture to thicken the sauce. Season with salt and pepper.

Combine the lemon zest, parsley, and garlic for the gremolata, and sprinkle a little over each portion just before serving.

chicken cacciatore

WLS ½ portion: Calories 151, fat 5 gr, carbs 7 gr, protein 15 gr
Serves 4

This was one of my mother's Sunday recipes. You can make this into a stew by cutting boneless, skinless thighs or breasts into 1-inch pieces. This recipe also works perfectly with a whole chicken, cut into serving pieces. Cutting the large breast pieces in half gives you 8 pieces of similar serving size. If you are not a carbohydrate watcher, serve this in a shallow flat bowl on top of a scoop of creamy polenta made with chicken broth and plenty of grated Parmesan. A tossed salad dressed with balsamic vinegar and olive oil completes the meal.

8 large chicken thighs, bone-in, skin removed, about 2 pounds

Kosher salt and freshly ground black pepper

2 teaspoons olive oil

1 medium sweet onion, diced

3 garlic cloves, chopped

4 ounces button or cremini mushrooms, sliced

1 medium green bell pepper, diced

One 14-ounce can crushed tomatoes in puree (see Note, page 122)

1 cup white wine or low-sodium chicken broth

½ teaspoon dried rosemary, finely chopped

1 teaspoon dried basil

½ teaspoon dried thyme

½ cup pepperoncini (Italian peppers) in vinegar, stemmed, seeded, and cut into rings

¼ cup black olive pieces (see Note, page 113)

Season the chicken with salt and pepper. Heat olive oil in a Dutch oven or large covered nonstick skillet over medium-high heat. Brown the chicken pieces and transfer to a plate. Drain off all but 2 teaspoons fat, and in the oil remaining in the skillet sauté the onion, garlic, mushrooms, and bell pepper until softened, about 5 minutes. Add the tomatoes, wine, rosemary, basil, thyme, and the browned chicken along with any accumulated juices. Cover, reduce the heat, and simmer 45 minutes, or until the chicken is tender. Add the pepperoncini and olives, and simmer an additional 5 minutes before serving.

pollo chile verde,
chicken stew with green chiles

*WLS ½ portion: Calories 141, fat 7 gr, carbs 7 gr, protein 14.5 gr
Serves 4*

This southwestern chicken stew was inspired by a dish I enjoyed
at a small trading post restaurant near the Grand Canyon. Use any
combination of green and yellow peppers but be aware of the heat
if you are straying from the varieties I suggest. Serve the chile
verde in a deep bowl with a drizzle of lime sour cream. I give my
family a large wedge of warm cornbread and they are very happy
people.

**8 large boneless, skinless chicken thighs, about 1½ pounds, cut
    into 2-inch pieces**
Kosher salt and freshly ground black pepper
All-purpose or Wondra flour for dusting
1 tablespoon olive oil
1 large sweet onion, diced
**2 Anaheim green chiles, Poblano chiles, or New Mexico green
    chiles, stemmed, seeded, and diced**
1 yellow bell pepper, stemmed, seeded, and diced
2 large jalapeño chiles, stemmed, seeded, and diced
4 garlic cloves, chopped
½ teaspoon dried oregano
½ teaspoon ground cumin
1 cup prepared tomatillo salsa or salsa verde (see Note, page 107)
Juice of 1 lime, 1½ to 2 tablespoons
½ cup reduced-fat sour cream
Grated zest of 1 lime

Season the chicken with salt and pepper and dust lightly with flour. Heat the olive oil in a large nonstick covered skillet over medium-high heat and brown the chicken pieces; transfer to a bowl. Pour off all but 2 teaspoons fat. In the oil remaining in the skillet, sauté the onion, chiles, bell pepper, jalapeños, and garlic until tender, about 5 minutes. Add the oregano and cumin, and sauté for 1 minute. Stir in the salsa, lime juice, 1 cup water, and the browned chicken pieces along with any accumulated juices. Cover the skillet, reduce the heat, and simmer 35 to 40 minutes, until the chicken is tender.

Blend the sour cream with the lime zest and juice and drizzle a bit over each serving.

chicken with tomato and feta sauce

WLS ½ portion: Calories 160, fat 8 gr, carbs 6 gr, protein 15.5 gr
Serves 4

I love feta cheese! It is tangy, fresh, and creamy with a touch of saltiness. I buy a large chunk at the local bulk foods warehouse store. My friend Constantine goes crazy for the Greek flavors in this dish. Serve with baby spinach sautéed in olive oil with garlic, and orzo pasta.

8 large boneless, skinless chicken thighs, about 1½ pounds
Kosher salt and freshly ground black pepper
All-purpose or Wondra flour for dusting
1 tablespoon olive oil
1 medium onion, finely diced
2 garlic cloves, minced

One 15-ounce can diced tomatoes in puree (see Note, page 122)

½ cup white wine

1 teaspoon dried oregano

¼ teaspoon ground cinnamon

4 ounces feta cheese, drained, rinsed, and crumbled

⅓ cup chopped pitted Kalamata or other brine-cured black olives (see Note, page 113)

Season the chicken with salt and pepper and dust lightly with flour. Heat the olive oil in a large nonstick covered skillet over medium-high heat and cook the chicken until well browned on both sides, about 3 minutes per side; transfer to a serving platter. Sauté the onion and garlic in the oil remaining in the pan until golden. Add the tomatoes, wine, oregano, and cinnamon, and season with black pepper. Return the browned chicken to the skillet with any accumulated juices. Cover, reduce the heat, and simmer 35 to 40 minutes, until the chicken is tender. Add the feta and olives to skillet, cover again, and simmer for 10 minutes more, until the cheese begins to melt into the sauce.

chicken paprikash

WLS ½ portion: Calories 162, fat 7 gr, carbs 9 gr, protein 16 gr
Serves 4

I am always trying new spices and ordering different varieties of the same spice to find new flavors. I order from Penzeys Spices—the on-line convenience has made it simple for cooks like me to try new varieties of old standbys. Some of my favorite discoveries are different varieties of cinnamon, vanilla, pure ground chili powders, curry powder, and for this recipe, paprika, all with different flavors and intensities. I order my Hungarian Sweet

Paprika from Penzeys, but there is a good brand, Szeged, that is available in most supermarkets. Spices quickly become dusty and flavorless, so be sure your paprika is fresh. For family and friends, serve over egg noodles tossed with butter and poppy seeds, along with some sautéed Brussels sprout halves.

8 large chicken thighs, bone-in with skin removed, about 2 pounds
Kosher salt and freshly ground black pepper
1 teaspoon olive oil
1 large sweet onion, diced
1 garlic clove, chopped
1 red bell pepper, cut into 1-inch dice
1 green bell pepper, cut into 1-inch dice
¼ cup Hungarian sweet paprika
½ teaspoon dried marjoram
½ cup white wine
One 15-ounce can diced tomatoes, drained
½ cup reduced-fat sour cream
2 tablespoons chopped flat-leaf parsley

Season the chicken with salt and pepper. Heat the olive oil in a large nonstick covered skillet over medium-high heat. Add the chicken and cook until well browned on both sides, about 3 minutes per side; transfer to a platter. Remove and discard all but 1 tablespoon of fat from the pan and sauté the onion, garlic, and peppers until softened and beginning to brown, about 6 minutes. Add 3 tablespoons of the paprika and the marjoram and cook, stirring constantly, for 1 minute. Add the wine, tomatoes, and the chicken pieces with any accumulated juices; bring to a boil, cover, reduce the heat, and simmer for 45 minutes, until the chicken is very tender. Remove the pan from the heat and transfer the chicken pieces to a platter. Blend the remaining tablespoon of paprika into the sour cream in a small bowl. Stir a large spoonful of the hot sauce into the sour cream and then blend the warmed sour cream mixture back into the sauce in the pot. Stir in the parsley. Add the chicken to the pan and coat with the sauce.

tandoori chicken

WLS ½ portion: Calories 100, fat 3 gr, carbs 3 gr, protein 15 gr
Serves 4

The yogurt in the marinade tenderizes the chicken and provides a creamy sauce to moisten the already very juicy meat. I serve this dish to my family with steamed jasmine rice and roasted asparagus spears. This recipe requires advance preparation.

8 large chicken thighs, bone-in with skin removed, about 2 pounds
½-inch piece fresh ginger, peeled and chopped
½ small onion, chopped
2 garlic cloves, chopped
½ cup low-fat yogurt
1 tablespoon Hungarian sweet paprika
1 teaspoon garam masala (see Note, page 129)
1 teaspoon ground cumin
1 teaspoon ground coriander
¼ teaspoon cayenne
½ teaspoon kosher salt
1 tablespoon lemon juice (about ½ lemon)
Vegetable oil cooking spray
½ cup low-sodium chicken broth

Make deep cuts 1 inch apart on the surface of the chicken pieces, slicing almost to the bone. Puree the ginger, onion, and garlic with the yogurt in a food processor or blender and blend in the paprika, garam masala, cumin, coriander, cayenne, salt, and lemon juice, to make a smooth paste. Pour the mixture over the chicken pieces in a ceramic or plastic bowl, turning to coat; cover and refrigerate 2 to 8 hours.

Preheat the oven to 450°F. Place the chicken pieces, coated with the thick marinade, in a lightly oiled baking pan and roast for 35 minutes, or until the juices run clear. Transfer the chicken to a platter and add the chicken broth to the hot pan, whisking to slightly emulsify the juices into a sauce, scraping up any browned bits. Pour some of the sauce over the chicken.

sesame roasted chicken

WLS ½ portion: Calories 151, fat 10 gr, carbs <1 gr, protein 14 gr
Serves 4

The sesame dressing used to marinate the chicken thighs is one of the most versatile sauces in this book. (This recipe makes about ¾ cup.) Keep a container of it in your refrigerator. For a quick lunch, I blend a tablespoon of the sesame dressing with one teaspoon of mayonnaise and mix it into a pouch of albacore tuna or chopped rotisserie chicken. I toss in a few handfuls of baby greens with a little of this dressing. Marinate game hens in some of the dressing before grilling, or drizzle it over roasted, sliced chicken. Use it on grilled or broiled seafood, too. Quickly sauté a pound of peeled and cleaned shrimp and add enough of the sesame marinade to coat for a simple salad.

Makes a great meal when served with Yukon gold mashed potatoes and baby greens dressed with some of the remaining marinade. This recipe requires advance preparation.

sesame marinade/dressing

3 tablespoons toasted sesame oil

3 tablespoons peanut oil

2 tablespoons soy sauce

3 tablespoons rice vinegar

1 tablespoon Splenda Granular

2 teaspoons whole sesame seeds

Freshly ground black pepper

8 large chicken thighs, about 2 pounds

In a small bowl, whisk together the sesame and peanut oils, soy sauce, vinegar, Splenda, sesame seeds, and pepper to taste until emulsified. Pour ½ cup of the marinade over the chicken thighs in a shallow bowl or plastic bag; set the rest of the marinade aside. Cover and refrigerate the chicken for 2 to 8 hours.

Preheat the oven to 425°F. Arrange the marinated chicken pieces in a small shallow pan skin side up, and roast 30 to 35 minutes, until the juices run clear when pierced with the tip of a knife. Drizzle a little of the reserved marinade over the chicken just before serving.

orange teriyaki game hens

WLS ½ portion: Calories 186, fat 5 gr, carbs 9 gr, protein 25 gr
Serves 4

Game hens are very moist and juicy, an ideal protein food for post-surgery diners. These birds are particularly succulent after an overnight soak in this Asian-flavored marinade. For hearty eaters, double the marinade and serve a whole hen to each person. This recipe requires advance preparation.

For guests, pair the hens with wasabi mashed potatoes and

sautéed snow peas. To make the wasabi potatoes, blend boiled
and riced Yukon gold potatoes with butter, milk, salt and pepper
to taste, sliced green onions (scallions), and a tablespoon of
prepared wasabi paste.

¾ **cup orange juice**
3 tablespoons soy sauce
¼ **cup Smucker's Light Sugar Free Apricot Preserves**
2 tablespoons toasted sesame oil
2 garlic cloves, minced
1 tablespoon grated fresh ginger
Two 20- to 24-ounce Cornish game hens, split in half

Blend together the orange juice, soy sauce, preserves, sesame oil, garlic, and ginger and pour over the hens in a shallow bowl or plastic bag.
Cover and refrigerate 2 to 24 hours, preferably overnight.

Preheat the oven to 400°F. Drain the hens, reserving the marinade;
arrange in a baking dish skin side up and roast 35 to 40 minutes, until
the juices run clear and the skin is golden. Reduce the reserved marinade in a small saucepan over medium-high heat until a thick glaze
forms. Drizzle a little glaze over the roasted hens just before serving.

grandma's lemon game hens

WLS ½ portion: Calories 269, fat 16 gr, carbs 1.5 gr,
protein 24 gr
Serves 4

My Grandma Helen makes the most delicious, juicy roasted
lemon- and oregano-flavored hens you have ever tasted. She
doesn't measure anything of course, so I had to watch her half a
dozen times to get the right proportions. For those not watching

their carbohydrate intake, mashed potatoes taste wonderful
mixed with some of the lemon sauce. Add a tossed salad dressed
with balsamic vinegar and olive oil.

½ cup lemon juice (about 4 lemons)
¼ cup olive oil
2 teaspoons balsamic vinegar
2 garlic cloves, minced
1 teaspoon dried oregano
Kosher salt and freshly ground black pepper
Two 20- to 24-ounce Cornish game hens, split in half
¼ cup chopped flat-leaf parsley

Preheat the oven to 425°F. In a large bowl, whisk together the lemon
juice, olive oil, vinegar, garlic, and oregano, and season with salt and
pepper. Loosen the skin on the hens but do not remove. Toss the hens
with the lemon dressing; arrange skin side up in a shallow roasting
pan. Pour all of the dressing from the bowl over the hens. Roast for 30
to 35 minutes, basting after 15 minutes, until the juices run clear and
the skin is nicely browned. Transfer the hens to a serving platter and
pour the lemon sauce and juices into a small saucepan. Bring the sauce
to a boil and reduce until slightly thickened. Stir in the parsley, spoon
a little sauce over the game hens, and serve the rest in a small bowl for
pouring at the table.

turkey tenderloins with creamy roasted garlic vegetable sauté

WLS portion, 3½ ounces: Calories 225, fat 8 gr, carbs 5 gr, protein 32 gr
Serves 4

What was I thinking when I ordered an entire case of garlic from an Oregon farm? For a week, I experimented with roasted garlic until I came up with the perfect recipe. My husband loves to dig into a bowl of this dip with my homemade baked spiced pita chips. I cut pita rounds into wedges, lightly brush the pieces with olive oil, sprinkle them with chipotle chile powder and salt, and bake them at 350°F until golden brown and crisp. Combined with sautéed zucchini and red peppers, the resulting creamy vegetable salsa is equally good on a piece of roasted mahimahi.

1 whole large bulb garlic

2 turkey tenderloins, about 1½ pounds

2 teaspoons olive oil, plus extra to coat the tenderloins

Kosher salt and freshly ground black pepper

4 ounces (¼ pound) reduced-fat cream cheese

¼ cup reduced-fat sour cream

2 tablespoons chopped roasted red peppers

2 green onions (scallions), thinly sliced, including green tops

¼ teaspoon dried thyme

¼ teaspoon dried basil

½ teaspoon Worcestershire sauce

3 medium zucchini, cut lengthwise into planks, then diced

1 small red bell pepper, cut into ½ inch dice

Preheat the oven to 400°F. Tightly wrap the entire garlic bulb in foil and roast for 1 hour. Remove the garlic from the oven and loosen the foil. When cool enough to handle, squeeze the roasted garlic from each clove into a small bowl and set aside.

Rub the turkey tenderloins with olive oil, season with salt and pepper, and roast in a shallow baking pan at 400°F for 30 to 45 minutes, until the juices run clear and the meat reaches an internal temperature of 160°F on an instant-read thermometer.

Puree the roasted garlic, cream cheese, sour cream, roasted peppers, green onions, thyme, basil, and Worcestershire in a blender or food processor until creamy; add salt and pepper to taste. Heat 2 teaspoons olive oil in a nonstick skillet over medium-high heat and sauté the zucchini and red pepper until very tender and starting to brown, 5 to 6 minutes; remove from heat, add the creamy roasted garlic mixture, and fold it into the vegetables as it melts. Thinly slice the roasted tenderloins and spoon on some of the creamy roasted garlic vegetable sauté.

achiote-roasted turkey breast with chimichurri sauce

WLS portion, 3½ ounces: Calories 80, fat 4 gr, carbs <1 gr, protein 22 gr
Serves 6

This entrée, inspired by a dish native to the Maya of the Yucatán Peninsula, uses a bright orange seed called *annatto*, blended with citrus and other spices, as a marinade. The authentic dish is wrapped in banana leaves and steamed over a wood fire—a bit difficult to duplicate in home kitchens (but worth seeking out when you visit the Yucatán). The chimichurri is a common accompaniment to sautéed, roasted, and grilled meats in Central and South America and is a fresh salsa that perfectly moistens the marinated, roasted turkey.

Although it is very simple to do yourself, you could have the butcher cut the meat from the frame of the turkey breast for you. This recipe requires advance preparation.

Juice of 1 orange, about ⅓ cup
Juice of 1 lime, 1½ to 2 tablespoons
7 garlic cloves
2 tablespoons ground annatto seed or achiote paste, a prepared
** version of annatto marinade available in the Latin or spice**
** section of most supermarkets**
½ teaspoon dried oregano
¼ teaspoon ground cumin
Pinch of ground allspice
1 whole canned chipotle chile, or 1 teaspoon Tabasco
** Chipotle hot sauce**
1 tablespoon plus ¼ cup extra-virgin olive oil
One 2½- to 3-pound boneless fresh turkey breast
½ cup loosely packed flat-leaf parsley
2 tablespoons red wine vinegar
2 tablespoons finely minced red onion
¼ teaspoon crushed red pepper
Kosher salt

Blend the orange and lime juices, 4 of the garlic cloves, ground annatto, oregano, cumin, allspice, chipotle, and 1 tablespoon of the olive oil into a spice paste in a food processor or blender. Loosen the skin on the turkey breast and rub the meat with the spice marinade. Lay the turkey breast out on a piece of wax paper, roll and tie with cotton string in several places to form an evenly shaped roast. Place the rolled roast in a shallow ceramic bowl or dish, cover, and refrigerate 4 to 24 hours.

Preheat the oven to 350°F. Place the turkey breast in a roasting pan. Roast to an internal temperature of 160°F on an instant-read meat thermometer, 45 to 60 minutes, until the juices run clear. Remove and set aside.

Pulse the parsley and remaining 3 garlic cloves in a food processor until very finely chopped; blend in the vinegar, red onion, crushed red pepper, and ¼ cup olive oil, and season with salt.

Thinly slice the turkey breast, arrange on a platter, and serve with the chimichurri sauce.

turkey burgers with muffuletta salad

WLS ½ portion: Calories 112.5, fat 8 gr, carbs 1 gr,
protein 10.5 gr
Serves 4

I used to make big, round, sourdough sandwiches with Italian cold cuts and a thick layer of this olive salad. In New Orleans, this sandwich is called a muffuletta. Although my big sandwich days are in the past, I wanted to use the same flavors of the salad as a condiment to moisten a burger. Adding shredded cheese keeps the burger from getting too solid and dry. My family enjoys their turkey burgers piled with the salad on a chewy sourdough roll, with hand-cut potato chips, while I eat mine without the bread with a little of the salad spooned over it. Also try this salad with broiled or grilled chicken, or roasted or sautéed fish. Lightly dust flounder fillets with seasoned Italian bread crumbs, sauté in olive oil, and top with the muffuletta salad.

muffuletta salad

  ½ cup finely diced artichoke hearts, canned or frozen (thawed)
  ¼ cup finely diced roasted red or yellow peppers
  ¼ cup pitted and chopped Sicilian green olives (see Note,
     page 113)
  ¼ cup pitted and chopped oil-cured black olives
  1 garlic clove, minced
  ¼ cup chopped flat-leaf parsley
  2 tablespoons olive oil
  2 teaspoons balsamic vinegar
  Juice of ½ lemon, about 1 tablespoon
  Kosher salt and freshly ground black pepper

turkey burgers

  1 pound lean ground turkey
  1 egg, lightly beaten
  ½ cup packaged Italian bread crumbs
  ½ cup shredded Cheddar cheese

In a large bowl, combine the artichokes, peppers, olives, garlic, parsley, olive oil, vinegar, and lemon juice; season with salt and pepper, and set aside.

Preheat the grill or broiler. Mix the turkey, egg, bread crumbs, and cheese in a large bowl, using your hands to combine gently. Shape into four ½-inch-thick patties. Grill or broil the patties until cooked through but still moist, 3 to 4 minutes per side. Serve with a little of the marinated salad piled on top of each burger.

turkey mushroom meatloaf

WLS ½ portion: Calories 143, fat 7 gr, carbs 4 gr, protein 15 gr
Serves 4

This meatloaf is very moist, tender, and easy to eat. A classic
served with mashed Yukon gold potatoes and green beans for the
family. Early after my surgery, I would mash together a small piece
of the meatloaf with a spoonful of the pan gravy and a few green
beans; not a very attractive mixture, but it tasted great and had the
perfect texture.

2 teaspoons olive oil
1 medium onion, finely diced
2 garlic cloves, minced
8 ounces cremini, portobello, or button mushrooms, finely diced
1 slice firm white or wheat bread
1¼ pounds lean ground turkey
¼ cup coarsely chopped flat-leaf parsley
1 large egg
½ teaspoon kosher salt
¼ teaspoon freshly ground black pepper
½ teaspoon dried thyme

Preheat the oven to 350°F. Heat the olive oil in a nonstick skillet over
medium-high heat and sauté the onion and garlic until lightly
browned, about 4 minutes. Add the mushrooms and cook, stirring
occasionally, about 4 minutes, until the released liquid has been
reduced to a glaze. Crumble the bread into a small bowl, moisten with
½ cup water, and mash with a fork into a coarse paste. In a large bowl,
gently combine the ground turkey, bread, sautéed vegetables, parsley,
egg, salt, pepper, and thyme. Spoon into a loaf pan, 9 × 5 × 3, smooth

the top, and bake for 45 to 50 minutes, until the juices run clear and the internal temperature reaches 160°F, measured at the center with an instant-read thermometer.

italian meatballs

WLS ½ portion, 2 meatballs: Calories 110, fat 8 gr, carbs 10 gr, protein 17 gr
Serves 6

Three years ago when my father retired and moved to Florida, I revived our family tradition of the Sunday spaghetti dinner. Since my bariatric surgery, I no longer enjoy pasta because of the carbohydrates, and the texture and consistency do not agree with me. I substituted ground turkey for the first few months post-op as it is easier to digest, but now I am back to using equal amounts of lean ground beef and pork. My family enjoys their sauce and meatballs on a plate of perfectly cooked spaghetti or ziti, but I am perfectly satisfied with one or two small meatballs napped with a little sauce and topped with some freshly grated Parmesan. I also serve a crusty Italian loaf and a salad of baby greens, tomatoes, olives, and artichoke hearts, tossed with olive oil and balsamic vinegar.

meatballs

1¼ **pounds ground lean turkey**
1 **large egg, lightly beaten**
2 **tablespoons freshly grated Parmesan**
½ **teaspoon dried thyme**
½ **teaspoon kosher salt**
½ **teaspoon freshly ground black pepper**

2 garlic cloves, minced

½ cup coarsely chopped flat-leaf parsley

½ cup packaged Italian bread crumbs mixed with ½ cup water

1 tablespoon olive oil

sauce for italian meatballs and spaghetti

1 tablespoon olive oil

1 medium onion, diced

3 garlic cloves, chopped

One 28-ounce can crushed tomatoes

One 28-ounce can tomato puree

One 6-ounce can tomato paste

1 tablespoon dried basil

½ teaspoon dried thyme

½ teaspoon dried oregano

¼ teaspoon crushed red pepper

Kosher salt and freshly ground black pepper

Combine the turkey with the egg, cheese, thyme, salt, pepper, garlic, parsley, and bread crumbs in a large bowl until very well blended. Roll the mixture into about 24 balls, 1½ inches in diameter. Heat 1 table-spoon olive oil in a nonstick skillet over medium-high heat and brown the meatballs on all sides. Transfer to a bowl and set aside.

Heat 1 tablespoon olive oil over medium-high heat in a Dutch oven or deep covered saucepan. Sauté the onion until softened, about 4 minutes; add the garlic and sauté an additional 2 minutes, stirring constantly. Add the crushed tomatoes, tomato puree, tomato paste, basil, thyme, oregano, and red pepper. Season with salt and pepper. Stir in 1 cup water, bring to a boil, reduce the heat to low, and simmer 45 minutes, stirring occasionally. Add the meatballs, along with any accumulated juices from the bowl, cover, and simmer an additional 45 minutes. Ladle the sauce over the pasta and serve with the meatballs.

desserts

So many people think that their pre-op eating frenzy of chocolate cake and Häagen-Dazs will be the last desserts of their life. Our relationship with cake and ice cream is forever changed by our surgery, but we can have an occasional dessert as long as we watch our sugar intake. Since my surgery, I no longer live to eat, and my tastes truly have changed. Sweets taste much sweeter, and I don't crave Entenmanns's Ultimate Crumb Cake anymore . . . at least, not the entire cake. I still love food and flavors, but I am satisfied with a small amount. I savor each bite instead of thinking about another plateful. I don't make dessert every night, I don't make them even twice a week; I make them occasionally when we have friends over for dinner, or when my girlfriends come and we sit on my patio and talk all afternoon, or when I have prepared a special dinner, or when I just want to treat my husband and myself. Incredible sugar-free desserts for special occasions can still be a part of our lives after our surgery. When I dine in a fine restaurant I will have one small bite of my husband's decadent dessert, but at home I prefer to make something sugar-free.

I don't want to cross the line into "dumping" territory so I stay well under 10 grams of sugar in one serving of any food; usually I am in the 5-grams-or-fewer zone to be safe. At home I can prepare desserts that have essentially 0 grams of sugar. It is an added challenge to keep desserts not only sugar-free but also low in carbohydrates. Every recipe in this cookbook has less than 15 grams of carbohydrates—most have fewer than 10 grams per serving—and that holds true for the desserts as well. I baked the blueberry cheesecake to take to a friend's home for her Christmas sweets table and it was the hit of the holiday! No one could believe that my light and creamy dessert was sugar-free and low-fat.

Splenda is my sweetener of choice. It is made from sugar and it measures like sugar, but without the carbohydrates or calories. The granulated version is excellent in recipes where the sugar doesn't provide the framework for the dessert, such as custards, creams, and fruit sauces. Equal for Recipes is another fantastic product and I prefer its flavor in specific recipes.

The nutritional analysis for each dessert is for a full portion based on the serving size.

belgian chocolate cheesecake

Full portion: Calories 173, fat 4.3 gr, carbs 7 gr, protein 6 gr
Serves 12

A perfect dessert. The chocolate flavor of the filling is intense; the chocolate cookie crust gives it an added boost of chocolate crunch; and it's sugar free.

1 cup Joseph's Sugar-Free Chocolate Walnut cookies (bite-size) (see Note, page 194)
1 tablespoon salted butter, melted
1 pound reduced-fat cream cheese
6 teaspoons Equal for Recipes, or 1 cup Splenda Granular (1 cup sugar equivalent)
¼ cup reduced-fat sour cream
2 large eggs
1 large egg yolk

> **One 3-ounce bar sugar-free dark imported chocolate (Guylian,**
> **Gol D Lite, or Torras, see Note, page 194), broken into pieces**
> **and microwaved at 50% power for 60 seconds, or until just**
> **melted**
> **1 teaspoon vanilla extract**

Preheat the oven to 325°F. Place the cookies in a food processor and pulse with the butter until you have moist, fine crumbs. Press evenly into an 8-inch springform pan or pie plate and bake 10 to 12 minutes, until the crust just starts to color. Cool on a rack while preparing the filling. (Leave the oven on at 325°F.)

Beat the cream cheese until smooth with an electric mixer; add the Equal, sour cream, eggs, egg yolk, melted chocolate, and vanilla, in order, beating thoroughly after each addition. Scrape down the bowl and blend again until smooth. Pour into the crust and bake 30 minutes, or until the center is barely set. Transfer to a cooling rack and run the thin blade of a knife around the edges of the cheesecake to loosen it from the springform pan (to prevent the cake from cracking). Cool to room temperature; chill at least 2 hours before serving. Serve small wedges with Splenda-sweetened raspberry sauce.

raspberry sauce

> **10 ounces frozen raspberries (Cascadian Farm 100% Organic**
> **Frozen Red Raspberries are so good and convenient that I rarely**
> **use fresh berries)**
> **¼ cup Splenda Granular, with additional to taste**
> **Pinch of table salt**
> **1 teaspoon fresh lime juice**

In a medium saucepan, bring the berries, 2 tablespoons water, the Splenda, and salt to a simmer over medium heat, stirring occasionally until the berries have softened and released their juice, about 2 minutes. Transfer the berry mixture to a food processor or blender and puree until smooth. Strain through a fine mesh strainer into a small bowl, pressing the puree through the strainer with a rubber spatula. Stir in the lime juice, and add additional Splenda if desired. Cover and chill.

Notes: Joseph's makes an excellent line of sugar-free cookies that are widely available in grocery stores. They are all natural and quite tasty. I keep several varieties on hand for sugar-free snacking and as a dessert ingredient. For a quick cream pie, I prepare a simple crumb crust using the cookies and fill it with cooked sugar-free pudding livened up with a dash of vanilla extract. A small chilled wedge served with a squirt of Reddi-wip is a great treat. Chocolate cream and banana cream pie are childhood comfort foods and my version is sugar free. The Joseph's Web site is listed in Sources, page 252.

The creaminess and flavor of these imported chocolate brands is remarkable, and they are becoming more readily available at grocery rather than just specialty stores. They can be ordered on-line and are listed in Sources, page 252.

blueberry cheesecake

Full portion: Calories 163, fat 12 gr, carbs 8 gr, protein 6 gr
Serves 12

Cheesecake is my ultimate holiday and special occasion dessert. You can either spread the blueberry compote on top of the cake for a beautiful whole cake presentation, or you can serve the cake in small wedges on dessert plates and spoon some of the topping over the slice.

1 cup Joseph's Sugar-Free Lemon cookies
1 tablespoon salted butter, melted
1 pound reduced-fat cream cheese
1 cup Splenda Granular
1 tablespoon vanilla extract

1 teaspoon fresh lemon juice

½ cup reduced-fat sour cream

2 large eggs

1 large egg yolk

blueberry topping

1 cup fresh blueberries, or frozen blueberries unthawed

2 tablespoons fresh orange juice

1 teaspoon cornstarch

2 tablespoons Splenda Granular

¼ teaspoon freshly grated orange zest

Preheat the oven to 325°F. Place the cookies in a food processor and pulse with the butter until you have moist, fine crumbs. Press evenly into an 8-inch springform pan or pie plate and bake 10 to 12 minutes, until the crust just starts to color. Cool on a rack while preparing the filling. (Leave the oven on at 325°F.)

Beat the cream cheese with an electric mixer until smooth; add the Splenda, vanilla, lemon juice, sour cream, eggs, and egg yolk, in order, beating thoroughly after each addition. Scrape down the bowl and blend again until smooth. Pour into the crust and bake 30 minutes, or until the center is barely set. Transfer to a rack to cool to room temperature.

Simmer the blueberries with 1 tablespoon of the orange juice in a small saucepan over medium-high heat. In a separate bowl, blend the cornstarch with the remaining tablespoon orange juice and add to the blueberries; stir constantly until the mixture comes to a boil and becomes glossy and thick. Remove from the heat and stir in the Splenda and orange zest. Let cool slightly while the cheesecake comes to room temperature. Spread the blueberry sauce just to the edges of the cake and refrigerate at least 2 hours before cutting and serving.

chocolate genoise

*Full portion: Calories 107, fat 7 gr, carbs 7.5 gr, protein 5.2 gr
Serves 10*

A moist cake with a tender crumb. The Dutch-processed cocoa gives it a deep, dark chocolate flavor. I serve it with just a dusting of confectioners' sugar. Take this basic chocolate layer over the top by making it into a sugar-free Black Forest Torte. Spoon a little sugar-free cherry pie filling over a wedge of chocolate genoise, dust the edge with confectioners' sugar, and top with Splenda-sweetened whipped cream.

The secret to making this cake is in the beating of the eggs. I use a medium glass bowl and set it over a saucepan of barely simmering water while I beat the eggs with my handheld electric mixer. The first time you make this recipe you will be amazed that you can whip eggs into a bowl of whipped cream-like silky foam. Be patient, as it does take 12 to 15 minutes. This cake must be refrigerated after the first 24 hours.

Vegetable oil cooking spray
½ cup all-purpose flour
**½ cup Dutch-processed cocoa (Droste is an excellent
    brand)**
6 large eggs, at room temperature
1 cup Splenda Granular
1 teaspoon vanilla extract
2 tablespoons salted butter, melted

Preheat the oven to 350°F. Spray the bottom and sides of a 9-inch round cake pan with cooking spray, line the bottom with a round of wax paper, and spray again.

Sift the flour and cocoa together into a large bowl using a fine mesh strainer and set aside.

Combine the eggs and Splenda in a glass bowl, beating with an electric mixer on high until double in volume, about 5 minutes. Set the bowl over a pan of simmering water to slightly warm the egg mixture, and continue beating for an additional 5 to 7 minutes, until the mixture is the consistency of softly whipped cream. Beat in the vanilla.

Lightly fold the flour and cocoa into the eggs, about one-third at a time, using a large rubber scraper and cutting through the batter, being careful not to deflate the mixture too much. Fold in the butter until just incorporated and pour into the prepared pan.

Bake for 15 minutes, or until a toothpick inserted in the center comes out clean. Cool for 10 minutes, turn out onto a cake rack, and carefully peel off the paper.

lemon–almond sponge cake

Full portion: Calories 129, fat 9 gr, carbs 7 gr, protein 6 gr
Serves 10

I didn't have a low-carbohydrate, sugar-free sponge cake to use as a base for my husband's beloved strawberry shortcake. So whenever I would indulge Ty, I ate just a few berries with a dab of Splenda-sweetened whipped cream. While I was experimenting with almond flour, using the principles for making a genoise, I came up with this moist, lemony cake. In addition to being a delicious cake to enjoy with a cup of tea, this it is the perfect base for my sugar-free strawberry shortcake. I slice a quart of ripe berries and puree ½ cup of the berries with ¼ cup of Smucker's Light Sugar Free Strawberry Preserves in a food processor, and then fold the puree back into the remaining berries. Spoon this compote on top of a thin wedge of the lemon–almond sponge cake and top with a generous dollop of Splenda-sweetened whipped cream.

You must use an electric mixer to whip the eggs. This cake can be made in advance and freezes beautifully as well. It must be refrigerated after the first 24 hours.

Vegetable oil cooking spray

¾ cup blanched whole almonds, or ¾ cup commercially prepared almond flour (see Note, page 199)

3 large eggs, at room temperature

¾ cup Splenda Granular

1 teaspoon vanilla extract

1 teaspoon lemon extract

3 large egg whites, at room temperature

¼ teaspoon cream of tartar

½ cup all-purpose flour

1½ tablespoons salted butter, melted

Preheat the oven to 375°F. Lightly spray the bottom and sides of a 9-inch cake pan with cooking spray, line the bottom of the pan with a round of wax paper, and spray again.

Using a food processor, grind the almonds into a fine meal; make it evenly ground, similar in texture to very fine bread crumbs. You should have ¾ to 1 cup of almond flour.

Combine the whole eggs with ½ cup of the Splenda in a medium bowl. Beat using an electric mixer until the mixture is the consistency of softly whipped cream and is triple in volume, about 12 minutes. Beat in the vanilla and lemon extracts. Using clean beaters, beat the egg whites with the cream of tartar in a medium bowl until soft peaks form. Gradually add the remaining ¼ cup Splenda and continue beating until stiff but not dry. Fold the whites into the egg mixture.

In a small bowl, blend ¾ cup almond flour with the all-purpose flour and gently fold into the egg mixture until incorporated. Fold in the melted butter. Pour the batter into the prepared pan and smooth the top. Bake 18 to 20 minutes, until a toothpick inserted into the center of the cake comes out clean. Cool 10 minutes, then turn the cake out onto a rack and remove the wax paper.

Note: I have recently discovered an excellent quality almond flour produced by Bob's Red Mill. It definitely produces results superior to my home ground almond flour so it is worth finding locally or ordering on-line (see Sources, page 252).

In addition, while shopping at the mall, I picked up a sunflower baking pan from Williams-Sonoma. It has transformed this plain sponge layer into the most beautiful sculpted cake you can imagine. I present the cake on a platter with decorative bowls of strawberries and cream. After the ooh's and ahh's subside, I cut a wedge of this lovely golden sunflower, and assemble each serving in a small dessert bowl (see Sources, page 252).

tangerine custard cakes

Full portion: Calories 130, fat 9 gr, carbs 7 gr, protein 5 gr
Makes six ½-cup servings

This light, tart dessert is the epitome of freshness and summer. Any citrus can be used for this tangy dessert. Sometimes I find fresh key limes in the market and will either use them solo or combine them with other fresh citrus flavors, but common limes, lemons, tangelos, and tangerines all add a tart flavor. The dusting of confectioners' sugar adds minimal sugar carbs but does make the dessert special, so I splurge without any danger of crossing the dumping zone line. This dessert also works well baked in a 1½-quart soufflé dish; increase the baking time by 5 minutes.

3 tablespoons salted butter, at room temperature, plus additional
   for the ramekins
⅔ cup Splenda Granular
Pinch of salt
3 large eggs, separated
3 tablespoons all-purpose flour
1 cup 2% milk
4 tablespoons fresh tangerine juice, about 2 small
   tangerines
2 tablespoons fresh lemon juice
2 tablespoons grated tangerine zest, about 2 small tangerines
Confectioners' sugar for dusting

Preheat the oven to 325°F. Butter six ½-cup ramekins and place inside a large roasting pan. Using an electric mixer, blend together the butter, Splenda, and salt until creamy and smooth. Mix in the egg yolks. Add the flour and milk and beat until well blended. Stir in the tangerine juice, lemon juice, and tangerine zest. Beat the egg whites in a deep bowl with clean beaters until stiff peaks form. Gently fold one-third of the meringue into the batter to lighten, and then fold in the remaining meringue until well blended. The mixture will have a somewhat curdled appearance. Spoon the mixture into the prepared ramekins.

Fill the larger roasting pan with hot water to come halfway up the sides of the ramekins. Bake 25 to 30 minutes, until puffed, lightly browned, and just firm to the touch. Carefully remove the ramekins from the water to cool. Just before serving, spoon 2 teaspoons of confectioners' sugar into a fine mesh sieve and sift over each of the slightly warm custard cakes. This dessert separates into a light spongy soufflé-like layer over a smooth custard layer and is delicious warm or chilled.

raspberry mousse pie

Full portion: Calories 147, fat 12 gr, carbs 8 gr, protein 2 gr
Serves 10

An intense berry puree whipped into a creamy fruit mousse.
This pie is a beautiful shade of soft pink. I have made it with
blackberries and strawberries but when I use plump raspberries,
I get the most applause. I am a raspberry fiend and a small slice of
this soft creamy mousse pie is the kind of dessert I dream of.

**1 cup sugar-free lemon cookies (Joseph's or Murray are
excellent)**

1 tablespoon salted butter, softened

1 pint fresh raspberries, blackberries, or strawberries

1¼ cups Splenda Granular

1 teaspoon unflavored gelatin (about ⅓ packet)

¼ teaspoon freshly grated lemon zest

½ teaspoon fresh lemon juice

¼ pound reduced-fat cream cheese

1 cup heavy cream

Preheat the oven to 300°F. Finely crush the cookies or pulse in a food
processor; blend with the softened butter and evenly press the mixture
into a 9-inch pie plate. Bake for 10 minutes and set aside to cool.

Puree 1½ cups of the berries with 1 cup of the Splenda in a food
processor or blender. Pass the mixture through a fine mesh sieve,
pressing on the solids to extract as much juice and pulp as possible.
Sprinkle the gelatin over 1 tablespoon cold water in a small cup and
set aside for 2 minutes without stirring. Warm the berry puree in a small
saucepan over medium-low heat, add the softened gelatin, and stir until
completely dissolved. Pour into a measuring cup and add water to the

berry puree, if necessary, to bring to ¾ cup total. Stir the lemon zest and juice into the puree. Beat the cream cheese in an electric mixer until fluffy; slowly add the berry mixture and beat until smooth. In a separate bowl, blend the heavy cream with the remaining ¼ cup Splenda and whip until medium peaks form. Gently fold half of the whipped cream into the berry mixture to lighten; fold in the rest of the whipped cream and the remaining ½ cup whole berries, and spread the filling in the pie shell. Chill at least 2 hours before serving.

lemon meringue pie

Full portion: Calories 128, fat 8 gr, carbs 10.5 gr, protein 3.5 gr
Serves 10

A lemon lover's classic and my father's very favorite dessert. He can't tell that this version is sugar-free and it just tickles me to see him taste it and try to detect if I am tricking him. The absence of sugar in the meringue keeps the whites from achieving a deep golden brown when baked, but a carefully watched minute under the broiler is a quick remedy.

1 cup sugar-free lemon cookies (Joseph's or Murray are excellent)
1 tablepoon salted butter, softened
1½ cups Splenda Granular
¼ cup cornstarch
¼ teaspoon table salt
3 large eggs, separated, at room temperature
½ cup fresh lemon juice (about 4 lemons)
2 tablespoons butter
1 tablespoon freshly grated lemon zest
2 drops yellow food coloring, optional

3 large egg whites, at room temperature
¼ teaspoon cream of tartar
½ teaspoon vanilla extract

Preheat the oven to 300°F. Finely crush the cookies or pulse in a food processor; blend with the softened butter and evenly press the mixture into a 9-inch pie plate. Bake for 10 minutes and set aside to cool.

Combine 1 cup of the Splenda, the cornstarch, and salt in a medium saucepan. Whisk in 1½ cups cold water. Cook over medium heat, stirring constantly, until the mixture comes to a boil. Reduce the heat to medium-low; continue cooking for 1 minute while the mixture thickens. Remove from the heat.

Whisk the egg yolks in a medium bowl to blend. Slowly whisk about a third of the hot mixture into the egg yolks, then whisk the egg mixture back into the saucepan. Return the pan to medium heat. Cook, stirring constantly, for 2 minutes, until the mixture is smooth and thick. Stir in the lemon juice, butter, lemon zest, and food coloring, and pour into the baked crust.

Preheat the oven to 275°F. Using an electric mixer, beat the 6 egg whites and the cream of tartar until frothy. Add the vanilla, then gradually beat in the remaining ½ cup Splenda, continuing until stiff peaks form. Mound the meringue on top of the warm lemon filling, spreading it to the crust edges to seal. Bake for 35 to 40 minutes, until the meringue is pale gold. Preheat the broiler and broil for 1 minute, watching constantly, until the meringue is browned. Cool to room temperature and chill before serving.

toasted coconut custards

Full portion: Calories 125, fat 8 gr, carbs 8 gr, protein 6 gr
Serves 8

A perfect coconut-flavored, smooth custard that is delicious
baked in a pie shell or in individual ramekins. I bake my ceramic
ramekins in a water bath for 30 minutes, or until the center jiggles
just a bit, and serve chilled.

Unsalted butter

**3 ounces unsweetened coconut (frozen grated coconut is
excellent; you can find it in the frozen fruits section)**

3 large eggs

**5 teaspoons Equal for Recipes (1 cup sugar equivalent), or 1 cup
Splenda Granular**

2 teaspoons coconut extract

1 teaspoon vanilla extract

3 cups 2% milk

**½ cup coconut milk, unsweetened lite preferred (not cream of
coconut)**

Preheat the oven to 325°F. Lightly butter a 2-inch-deep 8 by 10-inch
or 1½-quart round baking dish and place inside a large roasting pan.
Spread the coconut on a baking sheet and bake until lightly toasted
and golden in color, about 15 minutes.

Beat the eggs in a deep bowl until frothy and lemon-colored.
Gradually whisk in the Equal until well blended. Stir in the
coconut extract, vanilla, milk, coconut milk, and toasted coconut.
Pour the mixture into the prepared baking dish. Fill the roasting
pan with hot water to come halfway up the sides of the baking dish.
Bake 35 to 40 minutes, until the center is still a bit soft. Carefully

remove the baking dish from the water and let cool. Serve warm or chilled.

crepes suzette

Per crepe: Calories 67, fat 2.5 gr, carbs 6.5 gr, protein 2.5 gr
Makes 8 to 10 crepes

Make the crepes a day in advance if you wish—just stack, wrap in plastic, and refrigerate. The recipe also can be easily doubled or tripled to accommodate your number of guests. I usually serve two crepes per person for a light finish.

2 large eggs
½ cup skim milk
Pinch of table salt
2 tablespoons Splenda Granular
1 teaspoon vanilla extract
½ cup all-purpose flour
Vegetable oil cooking spray
1 tablespoon salted butter
¼ cup Smucker's Light Sugar Free Apricot Preserves
Zest and juice of 1 orange
¼ cup Grand Marnier or light rum
Whipped cream sweetened to taste with Splenda, optional

Whisk together the eggs and milk in a large bowl. Blend in the salt, Splenda, vanilla, and flour. Set aside for 30 minutes.

Spray a nonstick 8-inch skillet or omelet pan with cooking spray and heat over medium heat. Ladle 2 tablespoons of the batter into the center of the pan. Lift the pan from the burner and swirl the pan so the batter smoothly coats the entire bottom. Replace the pan on the burner and cook just until the batter looks dry. Flip the crepe, using a spatula or your fingers, and cook the second side for 10 to 15 seconds. Transfer to a plate. Repeat until the batter is used up, lightly coating the pan with the cooking spray between crepes.

Melt together the butter, preserves, orange zest, orange juice, and Grand Marnier in a large nonstick skillet over medium-high heat; gently simmer until the mixture comes together in a light syrup.

Working quickly, take the first crepe and dip one side into the warm syrup; fold in half, syrup-side in; and then fold again into quarters. Stack each of the folded crepes to one side of the pan while you prepare the rest. When all the crepes are folded, arrange them evenly in the pan and gently warm them in the sauce over medium-high heat for a minute, carefully turning each crepe to completely coat. Plate two of the warm, folded crepes on each plate, spoon on some of the sauce, and top with a little Splenda-sweetened whipped cream, if desired.

chocolate cream crepes

Per crepe: Calories 57, fat 1.5 gr, carbs 8 gr, protein 3 gr
Makes 8 to 10 crepes

This dessert was created for my weight loss surgery friend Stephanie, who moans when the waiter describes the chocolate selection from the dessert menu. You can get very creative with your choice of fillings but keep the carbohydrate count anchored in reality. I use my prettiest dessert plates and serve two delicate but richly flavored chocolate crepes rolled up around a filling of chocolate whipped cream and a few fresh raspberries, lightly dusted with cocoa and confectioners' sugar.

2 large eggs

½ cup skim milk plus 2 tablespoons

Pinch of table salt

2 tablespoons Splenda Granular

1 teaspoon vanilla extract

2 tablespoons Dutch-processed cocoa

½ cup all-purpose flour

Vegetable oil cooking spray

Chocolate Reddi-wip, or 1 cup heavy cream, whipped, and
  sweetened with Splenda and cocoa

1 teaspoon cocoa

1 teaspoon confectioners' sugar

Fresh raspberries or strawberries

Whisk together the eggs and milk in a large bowl. Blend in the salt, Splenda, vanilla, cocoa, and flour. Set the batter aside for 30 minutes.

Spray a nonstick 8-inch skillet or omelet pan with the nonstick cooking spray and heat over medium heat. Ladle 2 tablespoons of the batter into the center of the pan. Lift the pan from the burner and swirl the pan so the batter smoothly coats the entire bottom. Replace the pan on the burner and cook just until the batter looks dry. Flip the crepe, using a spatula or your fingers, and cook the second side for 10 to 15 seconds. Transfer to a plate. Repeat until the batter is used up, lightly coating the pan with the nonstick spray between crepes.

Place 1 crepe on a plate, make a thick line of chocolate cream down the center, and roll. Repeat with the remaining crepes. Place 2 rolled crepes on each of 4 plates. Spoon the cocoa powder and confectioners' sugar side by side into a fine mesh strainer and tap over the crepes to dust. Place the berries on the plate and serve immediately.

cream puffs

Per puff: Calories 74, fat 6.5 gr, carbs 2.5 gr, protein 1 gr
Makes twenty-four 2-inch cream puffs

This is a very simple dessert, and well worth the time it takes to properly prepare the puff shells. Using a food processor makes this a snap, as it takes strong arms to beat the dough without one. Resist the urge to pipe large mounds on the baking sheet, as they double during baking. Make them about the size of a cherry tomato for perfect three-to-a-serving cream puffs. Even though it is a bit unconventional, whipping the instant pudding mix with the heavy cream stabilizes the mixture and sweetens it as well. It is a delicious filling so don't discount it just because it uses instant pudding mix. The puffs can also be filled with small scoops of no-sugar-added ice milk and drizzled with melted sugar-free chocolate.

Vegetable oil cooking spray
2 large eggs
1 large egg white
5 tablespoons salted butter
2 tablespoons 1% milk
2 teaspoons Splenda Granular
Pinch of table salt
½ cup all-purpose flour
1 tablespoon Jell-O Sugar Free Instant Vanilla
   Pudding mix
1 cup heavy cream
1 teaspoon vanilla extract
Confectioners' sugar

Preheat the oven to 425°F. Lightly spray a large baking sheet with cooking spray. Lightly beat the eggs and egg white in a glass measuring cup; discard any excess over ½ cup and set aside.

In a medium saucepan over medium-high heat, bring the butter, milk, ¼ cup plus 2 tablespoons water, Splenda, and salt to a boil. When the mixture reaches a full boil, remove from the heat and stir in the flour with a wooden spoon until combined and the mixture pulls away from the sides of pan. Return the saucepan to low heat and cook, stirring constantly using a smearing motion, for 3 minutes, until the mixture is shiny and smooth.

Transfer the mixture to a food processor and process for a few seconds with the feed tube open to cool the mixture slightly. With the machine running, add the eggs in a steady stream, scrape down the sides of the bowl, then process for 30 seconds until a smooth, sticky paste forms. Scrape the mixture into a large plastic bag, push the paste into the bottom of the bag and cut off one corner about ½ inch from the tip to use as a pastry bag (or use a pastry bag if you have one).

Pipe the paste into 1-inch mounds on the baking sheet. Lightly smooth the surface of each mound using a fingertip dipped in water. Bake for 15 minutes, reduce the oven temperature to 375°F, and continue to bake 8 to 10 minutes longer, until golden brown.

Remove the baking sheet from the oven. With the tip of a small knife, cut a small slit into the side of each puff to release the steam, and return the puffs to the oven. Turn the oven off and leave the door ajar, drying the puffs for about 45 minutes. Remove from the oven, and when cool, store in an airtight container or plastic bag.

Place the pudding powder in a small deep bowl, add the cream and vanilla, and beat with a handheld mixer past the soft peak stage until the mixture gets very smooth and thick, about 3 minutes. Scrape the mixture into a large plastic bag, push it into the bottom of the bag, and cut off a corner about ⅓ inch from the tip. Just before serving, slice the puffs with a serrated knife, fill the bottoms with a swirl of the vanilla cream, and replace the tops. Dust with confectioners' sugar and serve immediately.

strawberry fool

Full portion: Calories 179, fat 15 gr, carbs 11.5 gr, protein 1.5 gr
Makes six ½-cup servings

This pudding captures the essence of fresh berries. I serve this dessert in a beautiful stemmed wine glass and spear a giant, whole, perfect berry on the edge of the glass for a dramatic presentation.

1 quart ripe strawberries, rinsed and hulled, 6 reserved for presentation
¼ cup Smucker's Light Sugar Free Strawberry Preserves
2 tablespoons Splenda Granular
Pinch of freshly grated nutmeg
½ teaspoon vanilla extract
1 cup heavy cream

Coarsely chop half of the berries and place in a small saucepan with the preserves and Splenda. Heat over medium-high heat until the berries begin to release juice and the preserves have dissolved, about 2 minutes. Transfer to a large bowl; stir in the nutmeg and vanilla, and chill. Slice the remaining strawberries and set aside. When ready to serve, whip the cream to stiff peaks. Stir the sliced strawberries into the cooled strawberry mixture and gently fold in the whipped cream, half at a time. Spoon into serving dishes and garnish with the reserved whole berries.

walker's favorite
chocolate pudding

Full portion: Calories 42, fat .5 gr, carbs 10 gr, protein 1 gr
Makes six ½-cup servings

One weekend I was experimenting with chocolate protein pudding recipes and it so happened that Ronni's sister Victoria and 3-year-old niece, Walker, were visiting from Seattle. At this particular time the mainstays of Walker's diet were bacon and chocolate pudding, so I obviously couldn't have dreamed of finding anyone better suited to judge which of the three versions was tastiest. I brought my three bowls of pudding to Grandma Joyce's house, and we had an old-fashioned taste test. This one was, without a doubt, Walker's favorite. She is now 4, and has since shunned bacon after discovering to her horror that it comes from pigs.

One 12-ounce package silken tofu
2 teaspoons vanilla extract
1 teaspoon Equal for Recipes, or ⅓ cup Splenda Granular
3 ounces sugar-free chocolate, preferably Perlege or Guylian
Heavy cream, softly whipped and lightly sweetened with
   Equal for Recipes

Puree the tofu, vanilla, and Equal in a blender until smooth and custard-like, scraping down the sides as necessary. Break the chocolate into pieces and melt in a small bowl in the microwave: heat on high for 45 to 60 seconds, until just melted. Add the melted chocolate to the tofu mixture; pulse until well blended and smooth. Pour into 6 individual dessert ramekins and chill. Serve with a swirl of whipped cream.

cannoli pudding

Full portion: Calories 123, fat 8 gr, carbs 6 gr, protein 8 gr
Serves 8

Once again the Italian in me comes to the surface. One of my "last meals" before my bariatric surgery consisted of anchovy pizza, with two cannolis for dessert. Little did I know that after my surgery I would be making cannoli cream that was indistinguishable from the full-sugar filling I have made for years. You must use a food processor to get the smooth custard consistency, because ricotta has a grainy texture that does not translate well into a pudding. This dessert should be assembled just before serving, or the pistachios will lose their crispness. Once you have shelled the pistachios, roll the nuts in a tea towel to remove the papery coating.

One 15-ounce container part skim ricotta cheese
5 teaspoons Equal for Recipes or ⅔ cup Splenda Granular
1 teaspoon vanilla extract
1 tablespoon sugar-free instant vanilla pudding powder
About 1 ounce sugar-free chocolate, such as Guylian,
    shaved
½ cup roughly chopped shelled pistachio nuts

Puree the ricotta with the Equal, vanilla, and pudding powder in a food processor until smooth and creamy. Transfer the mixture to a medium bowl and chill before serving. Place a swirl of the cannoli cream into a martini glass or small dessert dish and sprinkle liberally with the shaved chocolate and chopped pistachios; serve immediately.

fresh blueberries
with vanilla crème anglaise

Full portion: Calories 98, fat 3 gr, carbs 12 gr,
protein 5 gr
Makes four ½-cup servings

A great dessert for a hot day or after a comfort food meal when
you want just a little something sweet and refreshing. This vanilla
custard sauce is delicious with any fresh ripe seasonal fruit—
raspberries, kiwi, mango, blackberries, or strawberries are all
perfect for this presentation. Just watch the carbohydrate count of
your fruit selections; don't use more than one-third to one-half
cup of fruit to keep this dessert light. Garnish this dessert with a
single sugar-free butter cookie.

1½ cups 1% milk
Pinch of table salt
½ cup Splenda Granular
3 large egg yolks
1½ teaspoons vanilla extract
1 pint fresh blueberries, washed and drained

Whisk together the milk, salt, and ¼ cup of the Splenda in a medium
saucepan. Bring the mixture just to the simmering point over medium
heat. Combine the egg yolks with the remaining ¼ cup Splenda in a
medium bowl and whisking constantly, slowly pour in half of the hot
milk mixture, blending until smooth. Pour the egg mixture into the
saucepan, whisking until well combined. Place the saucepan over
medium heat and stir constantly until the custard is thick enough to
coat the back of a spoon, 5 to 6 minutes; it should never boil. Strain

into a bowl and stir in the vanilla. Let cool slightly. Place plastic wrap directly on the surface of the custard and chill before serving.

To serve, pile ½ cup of the blueberries in the center of each martini glass or dessert dish and pour the chilled cream around the berries.

coffee panna cotta

Full portion: Calories 102, fat 1.5 gr, carbs 12 gr, protein 9 gr
Makes six ½-cup servings

A quivering dish of coffee-infused cream. Add a tablespoon of Da Vinci Sugar Free Hazelnut syrup for a pudding version of your favorite latte.

2 teaspoons unflavored gelatin (about ⅔ packet)
2 cups evaporated low-fat milk
1¼ cups 1% milk
1 tablespoon vanilla extract
3 tablespoons ground coffee
½ cup Splenda Granular or 3½ teaspoons Equal for
  Recipes
Whipped cream sweetened with Splenda
Ground cinnamon

Sprinkle the gelatin over 2 tablespoons of cold water in a small cup and let soak 3 minutes without stirring. Heat the milks, vanilla, coffee, and Splenda over medium-high heat, stirring occasionally. As soon as the mixture starts to boil, remove the pan from the heat and add the gelatin mixture, stirring to completely dissolve the gelatin. Strain the mixture through a very fine mesh strainer into a large measuring cup. If necessary, strain the mixture several times to remove all of the coffee grounds, rinsing the strainer each time and allowing the mixture to settle before pouring. Pour into 6 ramekins or dessert cups. Chill 6 to 8 hours, until set.

To serve, run the tip of a knife around the edge of the custard, dip the ramekin almost to the rim into a bowl of very hot water for 15 seconds, cover with a dessert plate, and flip. Serve with a dollop of softly whipped cream to the side and lightly dust the entire dessert with ground cinnamon.

orange panna cotta with berry coulis

Full portion: Calories 110, fat 2 gr, carbs 15 gr, protein 8 gr
Makes four ½-cup servings

The tartness of the yogurt, the freshness of the orange zest, and the bright flavor of the strawberry sauce make this dessert a standout. Traditional panna cotta is a flavored cream thickened with gelatin, but this version has an unexpected burst of citrus. This dessert makes a nice presentation for a special occasion. I have little heart-shaped ramekins that I found at a discount store, and the white custard heart is beautifully contrasted by the strawberry sauce.

If you don't already have one, microplane graters are fabulous and this dessert gives you an excuse to buy one. One of these indispensable, super-sharp graters turns orange peel into a pile of golden gossamer threads that really infuse the custard with flavor.

1 pint (16 ounces) vanilla low-fat yogurt sweetened with
    Splenda or Equal, Blue Bunny Lite 85, or Dannon Light 'n Fit
⅓ cup Splenda Granular
1½ teaspoons vanilla extract
1 teaspoon freshly grated orange zest, lightly packed

2 teaspoons unflavored gelatin (about ⅔ packet)
5 tablespoons fresh orange juice
1 cup fresh strawberries (or unsweetened frozen strawberries)
2 tablespoons Smucker's Light Sugar Free Strawberry Preserves

In a large bowl, whisk together the yogurt, Splenda, vanilla, and orange zest. In a very small saucepan sprinkle the gelatin over 3 tablespoons of the orange juice and let stand undisturbed for 1 minute to soften. Warm the mixture over low heat until the gelatin has completely dissolved. Whisk the warm gelatin into the yogurt mixture and pour into 4 ramekins or custard cups. Chill the panna cotta at least 6 to 8 hours, until firm.

Place the berries, remaining 2 tablespoons of orange juice, and the preserves in a food processor or blender and process until smooth, adding a little additional orange juice if needed to make a puree. Cover and chill the sauce.

To serve, run a thin knife around the edge of each panna cotta, dip the ramekin, almost to the rim, into a bowl of very hot water for 15 seconds, cover with a dessert plate, and flip. Pour some of the berry coulis around each custard and serve immediately.

fresh cherry clafouti

Full portion: Calories 82, fat 2 gr, carbs 8 gr, protein 5 gr
Serves 10

This dessert is an amazing combination of fluffy, almond-flavored custard and sweet ripe cherries. The biggest, darkest fresh cherries are best for the ultimate flavor, but frozen cherries work well in a pinch if you drop them into the batter while they're still frozen. If you can't find cherries in the market, fresh or frozen blueberries will also make your mouth water. Once again, the

light dusting of confectioners' sugar will only add a gram or two
of sugar to the entire dessert, but really adds a spectacular
finishing touch.

½ cup 1% low-fat milk
½ cup part skim ricotta cheese
2 large eggs
½ cup Splenda Granular
½ cup all-purpose flour
½ teaspoon vanilla extract
½ teaspoon almond extract
Vegetable oil cooking spray
1 cup fresh pitted cherries
Confectioners' sugar

Preheat the oven to 425°F. Combine the milk, ricotta, eggs, Splenda,
flour, vanilla, and almond extract in a food processor or blender,
blending until smooth. Let the batter rest for 20 minutes.

Lightly spray the bottom of a 9-inch round ceramic baking dish
with cooking spray. Pour the batter into the dish and evenly arrange
the cherries in the batter. Bake 30 to 35 minutes, until puffed and
golden brown. Serve warm cut into wedges, and dust with confectioners' sugar.

spiced pumpkin custard

Full portion: Calories 84, fat 3 gr, carbs 8 gr, protein 6 gr
Makes eight ½-cup servings

Served warm with a dollop of whipped cream, this cinnamon and
ginger-flecked, creamy pumpkin custard is an anytime favorite. It
can also be an excellent addition to a holiday table, and a great

dessert to cart along to a family member's house so you can avoid the full-sugar pumpkin pie that is sure to be there.

Vegetable cooking spray
¾ cup Splenda Granular
½ teaspoon table salt
1 teaspoon ground cinnamon
½ teaspoon ground ginger
¼ teaspoon ground cloves
3 large eggs
One 15-ounce can Libby's 100% Pure Pumpkin (not pumpkin pie filling)
One 12-ounce can low-fat evaporated milk (not sweetened condensed milk)
Whipped cream sweetened with Splenda or Reddi-wip

Preheat the oven to 325°F. Lightly spray eight ½-cup ramekins or custard cups with vegetable cooking spray and place in a large roasting pan.

Mix the Splenda, salt, cinnamon, ginger, and cloves in a small bowl. Beat the eggs in a large bowl. Blend in the pumpkin and spice mixture. Gradually blend in the evaporated milk.

Ladle the filling into the prepared ramekins. Pour very hot water into the roasting pan to come about halfway up the sides of the ramekins.

Bake for 25 to 30 minutes, or until a thin knife inserted near the center of the custard comes out clean. Carefully remove the ramekins from the hot water. Serve warm or chilled. Top with Splenda-sweetened whipped cream or a squirt of Reddi-wip before serving, if desired.

light banana bread

Full portion: Calories 106, fat 5.6 gr, carbs 9.4 gr, protein 5.5 gr
Makes sixteen 1-slice servings

Everyone loves warm banana bread. This version doesn't have
any sugar and is light on fat as well. It was inspired by a recipe
from Canyon Ranch Spa that cut out most of the fat but not the
taste and with my simple substitution of Splenda, a few minor
adjustments of flavorings, and swapping whey protein for some of
the flour, this bread is sugar-free and even more delicious (in my
humble opinion). It does have a few carbohydrates, but with a
little planning you can still stay well within your daily intake
guidelines and savor a nice slice of this moist bread with a cup of
tea for a Sunday morning treat. Wrap and refrigerate this loaf as it
doesn't contain any sugar to preserve it.

Vegetable oil cooking spray
1 cup mashed ripe banana, about 2 or 3 medium
1 teaspoon vanilla extract
1 large egg
½ cup Splenda Granular
½ cup all-purpose flour
1 cup whey protein powder (I use ProPlete Gold Banana Crème
  Premium Whey Protein; see Sources, page 246)
2½ teaspoons baking powder
¼ teaspoon table salt
3 tablespoons salted butter, melted
½ cup chopped pecans

Preheat the oven to 350°F. Lightly spray a 9 by 5 by 3-inch loaf pan
with cooking spray.

Combine the bananas, vanilla, egg, and Splenda in a large bowl. Mix the flour, protein powder, baking powder, and salt in a small bowl and add to the wet ingredients, gently folding to incorporate. Add the butter and pecans and mix until just blended. Pour the batter into the prepared loaf pan and bake 40 to 50 minutes, until a toothpick inserted in the center comes out clean. Cool in the pan on a rack for 10 minutes, unmold, and slice with a serrated knife.

almond-anise biscotti

Per cookie: Calories 90, fat 8 gr, carbs 2.5 gr, protein 1 gr
Makes 2 dozen cookies

One of my nicest memories is of the many large tins of delicious biscotti my grandmother and her sister Lena baked at Christmas. When I started experimenting with almond flour, traditional Italian biscotti came to mind immediately, since most recipes already have almond extract and whole almonds in the dough. The result is amazing: toasted almonds, mild anise flavor, and the nuttiness of the almond flour—tough to believe it is sugar-free as well.

To really put these biscotti over the top, melt a 3-ounce bar of Guylian Sugar Free Belgian Dark chocolate in a shallow bowl in the microwave (45 to 60 seconds on high, then stir with a fork until melted) and dip the bottom of each biscotti, allowing the chocolate to come about ⅓ of the way up the sides. Place the dipped biscotti on a wax paper–lined baking sheet and pop the baking sheet into the freezer. When the chocolate is hard, transfer the cookies to an airtight container.

1 large egg

1 large egg white

1 cup Splenda Granular

2 tablespoons salted butter, melted

2 teaspoons vanilla extract

2 teaspoons freshly ground anise seed (See Note, page 222), or
substitute ½ teaspoon anise extract

2 cups almond flour (I use Bob's Red Mill almond flour, see
Sources, page 252) (or pulse 1½ cups, about 6 ounces,
whole blanched almonds in a food processor until it is
a very fine meal, resembling bread crumbs, and then
measure)

½ cup all-purpose flour

1½ teaspoons baking powder

Pinch of table salt

½ cup whole blanched almonds, toasted on a baking sheet at
350°F until lightly golden

Vegetable oil cooking spray

Using an electric mixer, beat the egg and egg white until thick and lemon-colored. Add the Splenda, butter, vanilla, and ground anise, and continue beating until well blended. Mix the almond flour, all-purpose flour, baking powder, and salt in a small bowl. Add to the egg mixture and stir until well blended. Give a few rough chops to the toasted almonds with a heavy knife, and fold them into the dough. Cover and refrigerate 20 minutes to firm the dough for handling.

Preheat the oven to 350°F. Turn the dough out onto wax paper that has been lightly sprayed with cooking spray and, using the paper, roll the dough into a 12-inch-long by 2-inch-wide flattened log shape. Transfer to a baking sheet by picking up the paper and rolling the biscotti log onto the sheet. Bake 35 to 40 minutes, until golden brown and firm to the touch. Cool completely on the baking sheet. Carefully remove the biscotti log to a cutting board and using a serrated knife, cut into ½-inch-thick slices. Arrange the slices on the same baking sheet. Bake 14 minutes at 350°F; turn the biscotti over and bake an additional 8 to 10 minutes, until golden brown. Cool and store in an airtight container.

Note: I have a small electric coffee grinder that I use just for spices.

strawberry italian ice

Full portion: Calories 42, fat .5 gr, carbs 10 gr, protein 1 gr
Makes six ½-cup servings

This dessert is simple, fresh, and fruity, with a hint of blended citrus. Substitute any unsweetened berry, or even fresh-frozen mango cubes for the strawberries; just use lower-carbohydrate fruits. Make a double batch for a backyard barbeque or outdoor party. The citrus syrup may be prepared in advance and refrigerated. It is also delicious as a sweetener and flavoring for iced tea.

One 16-ounce package frozen whole unsweetened strawberries
Zest and juice of 1 orange (about ⅓ cup juice)
Zest and juice of 1 lemon (about 2 tablespoons juice)
1 cup Splenda Granular

Slightly thaw the strawberries by placing them in a large bowl at room temperature while the other components are prepared, about 20 minutes.

Remove wide strips of zest from the orange and lemon with a vegetable peeler and scrape off any bitter white pith. Combine the Splenda with ½ cup water in a small saucepan and add the citrus zests and juices. Bring the mixture to a boil, reduce the heat, and simmer for

5 minutes. Allow the syrup to cool a bit, and then strain the mixture, discarding the peels.

Transfer the strawberries to a food processor or blender, add ½ cup of the citrus syrup, and pulse until a nearly smooth, frosty puree is formed, adding more syrup to blend, if necessary. Transfer the semi-frozen puree to a bowl and freeze 2 to 3 hours, until firm.

To serve, let stand at room temperature 15 to 20 minutes to soften slightly, scrape across the Italian ice with a large spoon, and place into serving dishes.

cooking for the holidays

Our fondest memories often center around holidays. We all have family traditions that make our celebrations special, and food is typically the basis of these customs. Most of us fear that our family holiday celebrations are over once we have had our bariatric weight-loss surgery. This is not true! The biggest change at my Christmas dinner table is that I was wearing clothes that were nine sizes smaller than the previous Christmas. It can be challenging, but with some planning and adjustments, we can prepare a fabulous holiday meal that we can enjoy every bit as much as the rest of our family and friends.

I was just 6 months post-op when my first holiday season rolled around. My first Thanksgiving celebration was a disaster because I didn't have control over the kitchen. The foods that my in-laws prepared were all wrong for me and I couldn't eat many of the dishes—they either had too much sugar or were too dry. When I returned home I was determined to come up with delicious holiday recipes so that my Christmas celebration the next month would be spectacular. Here are suggestions for Thanksgiving, Christmas, and holiday dinners and parties, prepared with love to celebrate the spirit of new health and happiness!

Holiday eating can be a problem for most of us. Pay attention to carbohydrates and watch for hidden sugar. I swore post-op that I would never prepare special diet meals just for myself. The changes that I have made to the menu to meet my needs are healthier for everyone at the table. So once again I am not the loner eating the soup!

Thanksgiving Menu

Thanksgiving is the most difficult holiday to reconstruct, as families have deeply ingrained food traditions and don't like anyone fooling around with their Mama's Pink Salad recipe. I have found that the best way to handle the feast is to make sure that among all the heavy carbohydrate dishes, there is some moist turkey, flavorful gravy, sugar-free cranberry sauce, and sugar-free pumpkin pie that I can eat. You can't eat much but you can enjoy it a lot.

roasted turkey

5-ounce portion dark meat: Calories 260, fat 10 gr, carbs 0 gr, protein 40 gr
5-ounce portion white meat: Calories 219, fat 4 gr, carbs 0 gr, protein 42 gr
Serves 8 with leftovers

For a postoperative person to enjoy this meal, it is imperative to have a perfectly roasted turkey. Just about everyone I know overcooks their turkey. An instant-read meat thermometer is key. Roast your turkey until the thigh reads 170°F and you will be astonished by the moistness of your bird. Even before my bariatric surgery, I would bring a meat thermometer as a hostess gift when invited as a holiday dinner guest. Brining poultry guarantees moist and tender meat; a kosher turkey has already basically been brined in the koshering and salting process, and is very moist and juicy.

One 12- to 15-pound kosher turkey, with neck and wing tips reserved for gravy, rinsed and thoroughly dried (Empire is a good brand)
2 tablespoons salted butter

2 teaspoons Bell's Seasoning
Kosher salt and freshly ground black pepper

Preheat the oven to 425°F. Melt the butter in a small saucepan and stir in the Bell's Seasoning. Place the turkey on a rack in a large roasting pan; dry the skin with paper towels, brush with the seasoned butter, and lightly season with salt and pepper. Roast for 1 hour; reduce the oven temperature to 325°F and continue to roast until an instant-read thermometer inserted into the thickest part of the thigh registers 170°F, 2½ to 3 hours. Remove the pan from the oven; carefully transfer the turkey to a platter and set aside for 20 to 30 minutes to allow the juices to be reabsorbed into the meat before carving.

pan gravy I

Per ¼-cup serving: Calories 47, fat 3 gr, carbs 3 gr, protein 1 gr
Makes approximately 2 cups

I always thought gravy was pretty important before having my gastric surgery, but now it is essential if I am even going to attempt to eat turkey. It is easy to make excellent gravy.

Turkey neck and wing tips, removed from the turkey after washing
   and drying
2 celery stalks
2 carrots
1 large onion, quartered
1 bay leaf
Several sprigs fresh thyme
12 whole peppercorns
2 cups low-sodium chicken broth
Pan drippings from roasted turkey

2 tablespoons cornstarch mixed with 3 tablespoons cold water
Kosher salt and freshly ground black pepper

Place the turkey neck and wing tips, celery, carrots, onion, bay leaf, thyme, peppercorns, and chicken broth in a medium saucepan, add 3 cups water, and bring to a boil over medium-high heat. Skim any foam that rises to the surface, lower the heat, and simmer for 60 to 90 minutes while the turkey is roasting, until the volume is reduced by half and the stock is flavorful. Strain through a fine mesh sieve, pressing down on the solids to extract as much liquid as possible.

Once the turkey is done and transferred to the platter, spoon out and discard as much fat from the roasting pan as you can, and strain the pan drippings into the turkey stock. Bring the stock and drippings to a boil and whisk in enough of the cornstarch mixture to bring the gravy to your desired consistency. Season with salt and pepper.

pan gravy II

Per ¼-cup serving: Calories 29, fat 0.5 gr, carbs 5 gr, protein <1 gr
Makes approximately 2 cups

When I roast a turkey breast and don't have the extra parts to make stock, I improvise and doctor up a packaged gravy.

1 tablespoon salted butter
½ pound cremini mushrooms, sliced
1 package Knorr Roasted Turkey Gravy mix
2 tablespoons dry sherry
½ teaspoon garlic powder
Kosher salt and freshly ground black pepper
Pan drippings from roasted turkey or turkey breast, optional

Heat the butter in a medium nonstick skillet over medium-high heat until foaming. Add the mushrooms and sauté until the released liquid has evaporated and the mushrooms start to brown. Prepare the Knorr gravy mix in a medium saucepan according to the package directions. Add the sautéed mushrooms, sherry, and garlic powder. Simmer for 2 to 3 minutes, until the gravy is bubbling hot. Add ½ cup of defatted pan drippings, if desired, to punch up the flavor.

southern style green beans

Per ½ cup serving: Calories 21, fat 0 gr, carbs 5 gr, protein 1 gr
Makes eight ½-cup servings

Green beans are low-carb, and when simmered the way my husband's Georgia family does it, albeit without fatback or lard, they are tender and incredibly delicious. The smoked turkey adds great flavor; most supermarkets now carry this product. I mash a few beans with my finely cut shreds of turkey for a moist mouthful. I don't make green beans any other way!

1 teaspoon olive oil
1 small onion, diced
¼-pound piece smoked turkey, cut from a wing or
  drumstick
1 teaspoon Cajun or Creole seasoning, page 133
2 pounds fresh green beans, cut into 1-inch pieces
Kosher salt and freshly ground black pepper

Sauté the onion in the olive oil in a covered saucepan over medium heat until soft. Add the smoked turkey, Cajun seasoning, and green beans; cover with water. Bring the beans to a boil, set the lid on the pan slightly ajar, lower the heat, and simmer for 40 minutes, or until the liquid is almost evaporated and the beans are very tender. Season with salt and pepper.

roasted sweet potatoes

WLS portion, ¼ small potato: Calories 40, fat 0 gr, carbs 10 gr, protein 1 gr
Serves 8

If you are going to eat carbs, make them count with good nutrition and lots of vitamins and minerals. I love sweet potatoes, and the silky, smooth texture satisfies my urge for potato. These salt-crusted roasted potatoes stay very hot while the turkey rests and you do your last-minute dinner preparations. To serve, cut a lengthwise slit in the potato and push the pointed ends toward the center, creating a pool for the butter and syrup for your dinner guests. I gild mine with a pat of butter and a drizzle of Steel's Sugar Free Country Syrup (see Note)—two bites of heaven. No one in your family will miss the pecan, brown sugar, and marshmallow topping, and they will all be healthier for it.

8 small sweet potatoes
Olive oil
Kosher salt

Preheat the oven to 400°F. Rub each sweet potato with a little olive oil, sprinkle with salt, and place on a baking sheet. Roast for 40 to 60 minutes, until the potatoes feel soft when the sides are pressed.

Note: Steel's Gourmet Foods produce a line of sugar-free syrups and preserves that are sweetened with Splenda or maltitol, a sugar alcohol that isn't absorbed or processed by the body so it has little effect on blood sugar levels. I have tried several of their products and think the Splenda-sweetened Cherry Pie Filling and the Sugar Free Country Syrup are excellent. (For information, see Sources, page 252.)

c r a n b e r r y   s a u c e

Per 2-tablespoon serving: Calories 10, fat 0 gr, carbs 4.5 gr, protein <1 gr
Makes approximately 2 cups

Make this a day or two ahead. No need for canned sauce when this sugar-free version is so quick and tasty. My husband prefers a smooth cranberry sauce, so I puree the sauce and pour it into a straight-sided glass to chill. To serve, I dip the glass into hot water for 20 seconds, cover with a dish, flip to unmold, and slice.

2 teaspoons unflavored gelatin (about ⅔ packet)
Juice and rinds of 1 orange (about ⅓ cup juice)
One 12-ounce package fresh cranberries
1 cup Splenda Granular

Sprinkle the gelatin over 2 tablespoons water in a small measuring cup and set aside for 2 minutes without stirring. Quarter the orange rinds. Combine the cranberries, orange juice, orange rinds, and ½ cup water in a medium saucepan, and cook over medium-high heat, about 10 minutes, until the berries pop and the mixture is very soft. Remove from the heat, remove and discard the orange rinds, and stir in the Splenda and the gelatin mixture until dissolved. Transfer to a decorative bowl or mold and chill several hours or overnight.

pumpkin pie

Full portion: Calories 113, fat 5 gr, carbs 12 gr, protein 3.5 gr
Makes two pies, each serving 8

Here's the famous Libby's label-on-the-can version with some adjustments. Sugar acts as a preservative in desserts; because this pie is sugar-free it *must* be kept in the refrigerator. This pie tastes like Thanksgiving and works for even the most recent post-op people.

2 cups sugar-free gingersnap cookies (Murray is a widely
    available supermarket brand)
2 tablespoons salted butter, melted
Spiced Pumpkin Custard (page 217)
Whipped cream sweetened with Splenda

Preheat the oven to 325°F. Place the cookies in a food processor and pulse with the butter until you have moist, fine crumbs. Divide the mixture and press evenly into two 8-inch pie plates. Bake 10 to 12 minutes, until the crusts just start to color. Cool on a rack while preparing the filling. Leave the oven on at 325°F.

Divide the pumpkin custard filling between the two pie plates. Bake 20 to 25 minutes, until the filling is set around the edges and the center is still a bit soft. Transfer to a rack to cool, then chill. Serve with a dollop of Splenda-sweetened whipped cream.

amazing pecan pie

Full serving: Calories 171, fat 14.5 gr, carbs 7.5 gr, protein 3 gr
Serves 10

The amazing thing about this pie is that it's sugar-free! The
ingredient list is specific, and substitutions won't work. To make
this pie you need Steel's Country Syrup, which can be ordered
on-line or by telephone (see Sources, page 252). When I tried to
make this recipe using other brands of sugar-free syrup, the
custard became muddy and, quite frankly, tasted awful. The Steel's
syrup is very thick, and that makes a huge difference. Even though
this pie is sweet, it doesn't have any sugar to act as a preservative
and must be kept in the refrigerator, or it will spoil quickly.

3 large eggs
¾ cup Splenda Granular
Pinch of table salt
1 teaspoon vanilla extract
4 tablespoons salted butter, melted
¾ cup Steel's Sugar Free Country Syrup
½ cup chopped pecans, plus 10 halves
One 9-inch homemade unbaked pie shell, not deep dish
Whipped cream sweetened with Splenda

Preheat the oven to 350°F. Beat the eggs in a large bowl until well
blended and stir in the Splenda, salt, vanilla, butter, and syrup. Mix in
the chopped pecans and pour the filling into the pie crust. Arrange the
pecan halves evenly on the custard and bake for 30 to 35 minutes, until
the sides are set but the center is still a bit soft. Cool to room temperature and serve in small wedges with Splenda-sweetened whipped
cream.

Christmas and Holiday Party Menu

I have put together this party menu, keeping in mind our food requirements. We can eat all of these foods but, more important, our guests will enjoy them as well. Every single item is a good food choice for someone who has had weight loss surgery—moist, easy to eat, and low in carbohydrates.

cocktail hour

Teriyaki Cheese Log with sesame flatbread crackers and crudités

Spiced Roasted Pecans

Ultimate Bloody Marys

dinner

Shrimp Louis Cocktail

Garlic-Herb Beef Tenderloin with Roasted Garlic Cream

Roasted Asparagus

Crisp Green Onion and Parmesan Polenta Cakes

dessert table

Individual Almond-Crusted Cheesecakes with Black Cherry
   Compote

Eggnog

Coffee with Sugar-Free DaVinci Syrups

teriyaki cheese log

WLS portion 1 tablespoon: Calories 50, fat 4 gr, carbs 2 gr, protein 2 gr
Makes about 1 cup spread

This simple and delicious cheese dip is excellent party food. Surround the log with sesame flatbread crackers and cucumber slices and garnish with green onion brushes.

½ pound reduced-fat cream cheese, at room temperature
1 tablespoon grated fresh ginger
3 green onions (scallions), minced
½ teaspoon garlic powder
1 tablespoon soy sauce
Sesame seeds

In a large bowl, beat together the cream cheese, ginger, green onions, garlic powder, and soy sauce until thoroughly combined. Chill until firm, 30 to 40 minutes. Transfer the mixture to a piece of waxed paper and roll into a log shape. Spread the sesame seeds in a shallow dish, then place the cheese log on the seeds and roll to coat. Wrap and chill until ready to serve.

spiced roasted pecans

Per serving, 6 to 8 nuts: Calories 54, fat 2.5 gr, carbs 1 gr,
protein <1 gr
Makes 2 cups

These toasted nuts are addictive. Since Ty's family lives in the
heart of a prime pecan-growing region, I always keep a supply on
hand in my freezer. I make this recipe in large batches and pack
them in decorative tins for holiday gifts or hostess gifts.

2 tablespoons salted butter
1 teaspoon Worcestershire sauce
½ teaspoon garlic powder
½ teaspoon Tabasco sauce
2 tablespoons Steel's Sugar Free Country Syrup, or 2 tablespoons
  Splenda Granular
2 cups unbroken pecan halves
Kosher salt

Preheat the oven to 300°F. Melt the butter in a small saucepan and stir
in the Worcestershire, garlic powder, Tabasco, and syrup. Pour over
the pecans in a medium bowl and toss to evenly coat. Spread the nuts
in a single layer on a baking sheet, generously sprinkle with salt, and
bake, stirring occasionally, until the nuts are crisp and toasted, 20 to
25 minutes. Cool the pecans on the baking sheet, breaking up any that
stick together. Store in an airtight container.

ultimate bloody marys

Full portion: Calories 80, fat 0 gr, carbs 4 gr, protein<1 gr
Makes enough spice paste for 20 cocktails

Many of us have questions about whether or not to drink alcoholic beverages after our bariatric surgery. You shouldn't even consider having a drink of alcohol unless you have discussed it with your surgeon and have his or her approval. With the new configuration of our organs, alcohol doesn't get a chance to digest in our tiny stomach pouch before being dumped into our intestines for absorption; this increases the amount of alcohol entering our bloodstream. In a nutshell, we must always be careful when drinking any alcohol as its effects are greatly amplified. After bariatric surgery we are cheap dates.

We must also watch our sugar levels and avoid carbonation. Most cocktails and mixed drinks use sugary mixers or sweetened fruit puree bases, and would quickly make us sick. Carbonation creates discomfort as our egg-sized stomach quickly fills with foam, causing us to belch after each tiny sip. When I was one-year post-op, I would occasionally sip on a wine spritzer, made from a little white wine with club soda, orange and lime slices, and lots of ice to dilute the carbonation. I love Margaritas but until I figure out how to make a sugar-free version using Splenda, they are off the list.

I occasionally indulge in my favorite Bloody Mary. I serve these tasty drinks at my patio brunches, and have included them in my holiday party menu as a cocktail hour drink. There is no sugar and no carbonation, and they still taste great with a half-ounce portion of vodka. If you skip the vodka altogether, you have a Virgin Bloody Mary.

1 cup grated prepared horseradish

2 tablespoons A.1. Steak Sauce

2 tablespoons Worcestershire sauce

1½ tablespoons Tabasco sauce

1 tablespoon celery salt

1½ teaspoons coarsely ground black
    pepper

1 tablespoon fresh lemon juice

1 tablespoon chipotle chile powder, or 1 tablespoon
    Tabasco Chipotle hot sauce

Absolut Peppar Vodka

Tomato juice

Lemon slices

Green olives

Blend the horseradish, A.1., Worcestershire, Tabasco, celery salt, pepper, lemon juice, and chipotle powder in a medium bowl until smooth. Combine 1 tablespoon of the spice paste with 1 ounce of Absolut Peppar Vodka and blend with 8 ounces of tomato juice. Pour the mixture over ice in a tall glass and garnish with lemon slices and olives.

shrimp louis cocktail

WLS ½ portion: Calories 75, fat 5 gr, carbs 3 gr, protein 10 gr
Serves 8

Be gentle when you coat the shrimp mixture with the sauce—the avocado cubes will mash if you are too aggressive. Use a large silicone spatula to carefully fold in the ingredients.

½ cup light mayonnaise

¼ cup bottled chili sauce

1 garlic clove, mashed with a pinch of salt

1 tablespoon fresh lime juice

1 teaspoon Tabasco sauce

Kosher salt and freshly ground black pepper

1½ pounds large shrimp, lightly poached, peeled, and
   deveined

1 medium Hass avocado, peeled and cut into ½-inch
   cubes

2 tablespoons minced red onion

2 cups watercress, trimmed, washed, and thoroughly
   dried

2 green onions (scallions), thinly sliced

2 hard-cooked eggs, quartered

Lime slices

In a large bowl, whisk together the mayonnaise, chili sauce, garlic, lime juice, and Tabasco until smooth; season with salt and pepper. Gently toss the shrimp, avocado, and red onion with about two-thirds of the sauce. Place a small bed of watercress in each of 8 large martini glasses or serving plates, and place a scoop of the shrimp mixture on top. Drizzle with some of the remaining sauce, sprinkle with the green onion slices, and garnish with a wedge of egg and a slice of lime.

garlic–herb beef tenderloin with roasted garlic cream

Per 3½ ounce portion: Calories 200, fat 12 gr, carbs 1 gr, protein 22 gr
Serves 8 to 10

Beef tenderloin is a perfect party or special occasion entrée; it is simple to season, effortless to roast to the perfect degree of doneness, and uncomplicated to carve.

2 whole garlic bulbs
1 whole fillet of beef (tenderloin), 3½ to 4 pounds
3 garlic cloves
2 tablespoons fresh rosemary, leaves only
2 tablespoons fresh thyme, leaves only
2 medium shallots
Kosher salt and freshly ground black pepper
2 tablespoons olive oil
1 cup reduced-fat sour cream

Preheat the oven to 400°F. Wrap the 2 whole garlic bulbs in foil and roast until soft, 45 to 60 minutes. Remove from the oven, unwrap, and set aside to cool.

Trim the tenderloin of excess fat and any tough outer silverskin. Tuck the thinner, tapered tip under the roast and firmly tie the entire tenderloin with cotton butcher's string at 2-inch intervals.

Turn the oven up to 425°F. Make an herb paste by combining the raw garlic cloves, rosemary, thyme, shallots, 1½ teaspoons salt, 2 teaspoons coarsely ground black pepper, and the olive oil in a food processor. Place the tenderloin in a heavy roasting pan and evenly coat the roast with the herb paste. Roast to an internal temperature of 125°F for perfect medium-rare doneness, 30 to 35 minutes. Remove the tenderloin from the oven and allow the meat to rest for at least 20 to 30 minutes before carving into slices.

When the roasted garlic is cool enough to handle, squeeze the garlic from each clove into a small bowl, blending into a smooth puree. Blend in the sour cream and season with salt and plenty of black pepper. Serve the herbed beef tenderloin at room temperature with the sauce.

roasted asparagus

Per 4-spear portion: Calories 15, fat 2 gr, carbs 3 gr, protein 1 gr
Serves 8

Roasting asparagus intensifies its flavor, and makes the spears
easy to eat.

2 pounds fresh asparagus, bottoms trimmed and peeled
1 tablespoon olive oil
1 teaspoon balsamic vinegar
Kosher salt and freshly ground black pepper

Preheat the oven to 500°F. Toss the asparagus with the olive oil and vinegar in a large bowl, and place them in a single layer on a baking sheet. Season with salt and pepper. Roast for 12 minutes, or until the asparagus are tender when pierced with the tip of a knife, but still firm. Transfer to a serving platter.

crisp green onion
and parmesan polenta cakes

WLS ½ portion: Calories 60, fat 3.5 gr, carbs 7.5 gr, protein 1 gr
Makes 9 polenta squares

A perfect counterpart to the roasted tenderloin for the folks not
watching their carbohydrates. Now that I am over 2½ years post-
surgery, I will have a small portion of this delicious dish. If I am
going to have a carbohydrate, I want to be sure it is delectable.
Who wants to waste their precious few carbohydrate grams on
boring mashed potatoes? This dish can be prepared in advance
to the point of refrigerating the seasoned polenta mixture; leave
the cutting and browning of the cakes for last-minute preparation
while the asparagus spears roast.

2 tablespoons salted butter
1 cup stone-ground polenta or yellow stone-ground grits
  (see Note, page 137)
2 tablespoons olive oil
2 bunches green onions (scallions), thinly sliced
½ cup freshly grated Parmesan
Kosher salt and freshly ground black pepper
Vegetable cooking oil spray
All-purpose or Wondra flour for dusting

Bring 5 cups of water and the butter to a boil in a large saucepan over
medium-high heat. Slowly whisk in the polenta, stirring constantly to
prevent lumping. Reduce the heat to low, cover, and simmer, stirring
frequently, until the polenta is tender, about 30 minutes.

While the polenta is cooking, sauté the green onions in 1 tablespoon of the olive oil in a medium saucepan until soft, about 4 minutes. Set aside.

Remove the polenta from the heat, stir in the green onions and Parmesan, and season with salt and pepper. Pour into a lightly sprayed 9 by 9-inch baking pan, smooth the top, and refrigerate until firm, about 2 hours. Turn the firm polenta out onto a piece of plastic wrap, and cut into 9 squares.

Heat the remaining tablespoon of olive oil in a large nonstick skillet over medium-high heat. Lightly dust the top and bottom of each polenta square with flour, add to the pan in a single layer and cook until brown and crisp, about 4 minutes per side.

individual almond-crusted cheesecakes with black cherry compote

Full portion: Calories 196, fat 14 gr, carbs 10 gr, protein 7 gr
Serves 10

A fabulous pairing of almond and cherry shines in the perfect ending for this holiday feast. It is so simple to make these individual cakes in advance and keep them on a tray in the refrigerator until dessert time. No complicated serving preparations or cutting—just unmold and pour on a little of the cherry sauce.

1½ cups Joseph's Sugar Free Almond cookies, bite-size
1 tablespoon salted butter, softened
1½ pounds reduced-fat cream cheese, at room temperature
1¾ cups Splenda Granular

1 teaspoon almond extract

2 teaspoons vanilla extract

½ cup reduced-fat sour cream

3 large eggs plus 1 additional yolk, lightly beaten

½ cup sliced almonds

2 cups pitted fresh black cherries, sliced (or frozen, unthawed)

2 teaspoons cornstarch

2 tablespoons amaretto

Preheat the oven to 325°F. In a food processor, grind the almond cookies until they are the texture of fine bread crumbs. Blend in the butter. Press a couple of tablespoons of the crust crumbs into each of 10 six-ounce heavy foil cups that have been lightly sprayed with cooking spray. Place on a baking sheet and bake 6 to 8 minutes, until the crusts just start to color.

Using an electric mixer, beat the cream cheese until smooth; add 1½ cups of the Splenda, the almond extract, vanilla, sour cream, and eggs, beating thoroughly after each addition. Scrape down the bowl and blend again until smooth. Fill each cup ⅔ full, place a few sliced almonds on each cake, and bake 18 to 20 minutes, or until the center is barely set. Place the baking sheet on a rack and cool to room temperature. Chill in the refrigerator at least 2 hours before serving.

Bring the cherries, the remaining ¼ cup of Splenda, and ¼ cup water to a boil in a medium saucepan; lower the heat and simmer. Blend the cornstarch with the amaretto in a small cup and add to the cherry mixture, stirring constantly until the mixture thickens and becomes glossy. Transfer to a small bowl and chill before using.

Unmold each cheesecake onto a dessert plate, and spoon on some of the cherry sauce.

e g g n o g

Full portion: Calories 80, fat 2 gr, carbs 6 gr, protein 4.5 gr
Makes 12 ½-cup servings

6 cups 2% milk
1 cup Splenda Granular
6 egg yolks
1 tablespoon vanilla extract
Freshly grated nutmeg
¼ cup dark rum or amaretto

Whisk together 5 cups of the milk and ½ cup of the Splenda in a medium saucepan and bring the mixture just to the simmering point over medium heat. Beat the egg yolks with the remaining ½ cup Splenda in a medium bowl and, whisking constantly, slowly pour in half of the hot milk, blending until smooth. Pour the eggs and milk back into the saucepan, whisking until well combined. Place the saucepan over medium-low heat and stirring constantly, cook until the custard is thick enough to coat the back of a spoon, 6 to 8 minutes; it should never boil. Remove from the heat and stir in the vanilla and ½ teaspoon freshly grated nutmeg. Cool slightly. Pour the mixture though a fine mesh strainer into a bowl or pitcher, cover, and chill. Just before serving, stir in the rum and the additional 1 cup milk, if necessary, to achieve the desired consistency. Serve in small glasses with a generous grating of nutmeg.

sources

When you first get involved in the process of having weight loss surgery, it can be overwhelming to wade through all of the information in order to figure out what you need in the way of protein shakes, protein bars, vitamins, and mineral supplements. I see so many early post-op people in our support group meetings and on message boards that are confused by the sheer numbers of products on the market and many end up choosing products that are not at all suitable for post-op bariatric patients. There are protein powders and bars out there that are extremely high in carbs and contain sugar, and then there are those that are appropriate for us by the numbers but simply taste terrible; we don't all need to repeat the same mistakes in buying them.

This is why I have created a companion website to this book where you can find the newest and best products that are within our specific dietary guidelines. Check back often to see what great products have been added in addition to new recipes and new information that may affect our health.

www.BariatricEating.com Toll free line: 1-888-777-4202

Nutritional Analysis
USDA Nutrient Database. Type in any food and see the nutritional analysis of protein, carbohydrates, fat, vitamins, minerals, and other components. This site belongs in your favorite places folder on your computer toolbar.

www.nal.usda.gov/fnic/foodcomp/index.html

Another superb source of nutrition and fitness information is located on-line at FitDay. It is an excellent place for you to keep a daily record of the foods you eat and the exercise you get. Based on your journal entries, this website analyzes your diet, exercise, and weight loss, and generates easy-to-read charts and tables tracking your short- and long-term progress. I love the "Today's Foods" section—I can add up every morsel I put into my mouth and get a total nutritional breakdown. There is no ignoring too many carbs or too little protein with this feature.

www.fitday.com

Low Carb, Sugar-Free and/or Protein-Rich Products
protein powder

Experiment with protein powders to find one that you like before you have your surgery. Do NOT choose a protein supplement that is high in carbohydrates; these formulations are for body builders, not bariatric weight loss people. Low carbohydrate content is crucial for us, so read the label and choose a powder that contains no more than 5 grams of carbs per shake and has at least 20 to 30 grams of protein per scoop.

ProPlete Gold from **Labrada** makes the best protein shakes I have tasted. The fruit flavors contain dried pieces of fruit and the chocolate is rich and flavorful. One scoop of Banana Crème with 4 ounces of low-fat milk or water and a little ice shakes up into a smooth delicious shake in 30 seconds; plus it is sugar-free and low carb. This is the protein powder that I use in my Light Banana Bread recipe with unbelievable results.

Labrada *ProPlete Gold Complete Whey Protein* www.Labrada. com, www.BariatricEating.com

Nectar from SYNTRAX, Fruit Juice Flavored Whey Protein Isolate is an excellent water-based protein drink. The flavors are a sweet-tart combination that reminds me of Jolly Rancher candy. A welcome addition to creamy milkshakes. www.SYNTRAX.com, www. BariatricEating.com

Zero Carb Isopure is a good-tasting protein powder. There are no off-flavors so it is an excellent base for great-tasting blender shakes. There are several formulations of Isopure, so make sure you choose the Zero Carb variety. This brand contains 0 carbs per shake, and each two-scoop shake pumps 50 grams of protein into your system.

Nature's Best Zero Carb Isopure Protein Powder www.Natures Best.com, www.BariatriceEating.com

Designer Whey, produced by **NEXT Proteins**, is another excellent product for bariatric patients. It has a good flavor and mixes up smoothly. I enjoy the vanilla praline for a light caramel-flavored shake.

NEXT Protein Designer Whey Powder www.designerwhey.com, www.BariatricEating.com

Optimum Nutrition's *Any Whey* www.BariatricEating.com is an instant, tasteless whey protein that melts invisibly into puddings, chili, and even Crystal Lite. I recommend these unflavored protein granules to add some extra protein to soups and savory foods. There are many people who just don't like to drink milkshakes, and the unflavored protein works well for them; they can stir a scoop into some hot chicken broth. This product contains 35 grams of protein with just 4 grams of carbs in a two-scoop serving.

EAS makes two excellent product lines that are well-suited for bariatric patients and our low-carbohydrate, high-protein needs: **AdvantEdge Carb Control** and **Myoplex Carb Sense**. I regularly use the AdvantEdge Carb Control ready-to-drink shakes. The juice box packaging is convenient, and the chocolate fudge tastes like chocolate milk. Keep a stash of these shakes in the refrigerator and grab one when you are on the go. When faced with a weekend trip or a vacation, the light four-pack carton fits in the corner of my suitcase; I pop them into the mini bar to chill them for a quick protein fix while getting ready in the morning. These are now widely available in grocery stores, so I usually pack one carton and buy additional shakes while on my trip. The EAS AdvantEdge Carb Control line is available at Wal-Mart and many large grocery chain stores.

EAS *AdvantEdge Carb Control* and *Myoplex Carb Sense* products www.Eas.com, www.BariatricEating.com

protein bars

Don't eat protein bars that are high in carbs and sugar! There are many formulations of these bars that are purposely high in carbs for body builders and athletes; these are NOT the ones you want. I see WLS patients eating Luna and Balance bars with 15 to 35 grams of sugar and it just makes me shake my head. No doubt they are delicious but they have sugar in them and are not for us. The low-carb bars are usually in their own section, have just 2 to 8 net impact carbs with 20 to 35 grams of protein, and taste great. "Net Impact" carbohydrates are calculated by subtracting the dietary fiber and other low glycemic carbohydrates (i.e., sugar alcohols) from the "Total Carbohydrates." Sugar alcohols can be deducted from total carb counts because they are not digested and do not impact our blood sugar levels. Be aware that commonly used sugar alcohols such as glycerin, maltitol, and glycerol can have a laxative effect on some people. Always read the nutrition facts label on a bar before buying it.

I am amazed by the changes in this product category in just the past couple of years that I have been eating protein bars. I used to look for the bar that was the least objectionable, and the choice was between chocolate-flavored clay and peanut butter–flavored clay. Today there are bars that are as delicious as a regular candy bar that are totally within our dietary guidelines. These are my current favorites.

Premier Nutrition *Odyssey Triple Layer Caramel Nut* **bar** could put Snickers out of business. Contains 4 net impact carbs and 30 grams of protein. These bars are better tasting than Detour and do not push the sugar limits into the danger zone.

EAS *Myoplex Carb Sense Marble Fudge* **bar** has a creamy cookie dough nougat studded with crunchy pieces of chocolate sandwich cookie. Contains 5 net impact carbs and 29 grams of protein.

Biochem *Strive Mixed Berry Crunch* **bar** tastes like a strawberry Rice Krispie Treat. The Chocolate S'mores is an amazingly good cocoa version. Contains 3 net impact carbs and 20 grams of protein.

Premier Nutrition *Protein 8 Chocolate Coconut* **bar** tastes like a chocolate coconut macaroon. Contains 1 net impact carb and 30 grams of protein.

The best on-line source for all of these protein bars is **www. BariatricEating.com,** as I constantly revise the list as new bars come into the marketplace.

Vitamins and Minerals

Because of potential vitamin deficiencies due to the small amounts of food we ingest, we must take vitamin supplements for the rest of our lives. VistaVitamins Wellness MultiVitamin and Mineral supplements have been formulated for gastric bypass surgery patients and not only contain everything that we need to maintain good health but also use chemical principles so the vitamins and minerals can pass through the intestinal lining to our tissues.

Chewable Wellness Formula—citrus punch flavored chewable wafers containing all the essential nutrients, including fat and water-soluble vitamins and amino acid chelated minerals. A special formula for pre-op and new post-op patients.

Wellness Plus Capsules—Convenient AM/PM packets of capsules containing all of the essential nutrients found in the Chewable Wellness Formula, plus increased concentrations of B vitamins and higher levels of amino acid chelated minerals. For digestive and immune system conditioning, specialized acidophilus and fiber ingredients are included.

VistaVitamins for Gastric Bypass Patients, www.VistaVitamins. com, www.BariatricEating.com

After weight loss surgery, we must remain aware of our calcium position so that we don't suffer from osteoporosis later in life. I take Vista-Vitamins so that I do not need to take a separate calcium supplement but if your surgeon has a different vitamin-mineral regime and you need a good calcium citrate supplement, Tropical Oasis makes a liquid that provides our daily required dose in just one tasty tablespoon.

Tropical Oasis *Liquid Calcium Magnesium* www.TropicalOasis. com

Grocery Items

If you have trouble locating some of the recipe components in your area, one of the best on-line sources for distinctive and unusual ingredients is Ethnic Grocer. Products are organized so you can shop by country or by category to make it easy to find that special ingredient that makes the dish. Here are some of my favorite ingredients.

www.EthnicGrocer.com

Tahini: ground sesame paste

Kalamata olives: brine-cured black olives

Garam masala: Indian spice blend that may include cumin, black pepper, cinnamon, cloves, coriander, and cardamon.

Ancho chiles: spicy, sweet raisin-like flavored, medium-hot chile, available whole or ground

Guajillo chiles: flavorful hot chile, available whole, dried

Coconut milk: unsweetened liquid pressed from grated coconuts

Chipotle peppers: smoked, dried red jalapeño, available canned in adobo sauce or ground

Wasabi: pungent Japanese variety of horseradish, available either dried or as a prepared paste

Hoisin sauce: Chinese sauce with a sweet-smoky flavor

Sushi ginger: thinly sliced ginger packed in sweetened vinegar; this Japanese accompaniment is also called *gari*

Sun-dried tomatoes: delicious concentrated tomato flavor, dried or packed in oil

Toasted sesame oil: mildly nutty and aromatic seasoning widely used in Asian cooking.

Annatto seed: often ground into a paste, and blended with vinegar and garlic, as a Mexican seasoning paste called achiote. Prepared achiote paste is a substitute.

The following are individual products that I happen to love. Most of them are available locally although you may have to hunt a bit for them. If you cannot locate them you can always order them from the source.

Di Vinci Sugar-Free Syrups are sweetened with Splenda, and add great taste to shakes and sauces. The array of flavors is incredible. **www.DaVinciGourmet.com,** 1-800-640-6779

Chef Rick Bayless's line of salsas, marinades, and sauces are excellent to use in recipes or as a simple condiment to moisten anything. I have at least four jars in my kitchen right now **www.Frontera Kitchens.com,** 1-800-509-4441 ext. 120

Napa Valley chef Micheal Chiarello's excellent line of marinades, dressings, and infused oils are flavorful and original. I am addicted to the fat-free Mango and Raspberry Balsamic dressings. **www.Con sorzio.com,** 1-800-288-1089

Muir Glen has a line of fire-roasted tomato products that add a smoky flavor to many of my braised dishes and sauces. **www.Muir Glen.com,** 1-800-624-4123

Penzeys Spices is the best source for spices and pure, natural extracts. Throw out those old muted tins and bottles in your cabinet and start over with fresh from Penzeys; you will not believe the difference it will make in the flavor of your dishes. **www.Penzeys.com,** 1-800-741-7787

The Nora Mill Granary in Helen, Georgia, has been in operation since 1876 and still uses a water-powered wheel to grind their grains. The stone-ground grits are absolutely delicious. **www.NoraMill.com,** 1-800-927-2375

For years I have reached for the Tony Chachere's Original Creole Seasoning in my kitchen. **www.TonyChacheres.com,** 1-800-551-9066

Steel's Sugar Free Country Syrup makes a perfect sugar-free pecan pie. **www.SteelsGourmet.com,** 1-800-6-STEELS

Joseph's Sugar Free Cookies are excellent for snacking and perfect for sugar-free dessert crusts. **www.JosephsLiteCookies.com,** 1-505-546-2839

Guylian, No Sugar Added Dark and Milk Chocolate are smooth, creamy, delicious Belgran chocolates. **www.BariatricEating.com**

Since I sometimes have a difficult time finding a consistant local source for imported sugar-free chocolate for my recipes, I have both Gol D Lite Sugar Free Belgian chocolate and Torras Sugar Free Spanish chocolate available on my website. **www.BariatricEating.com,** 1-888-777-4202

Williams-Sonoma continues to be one of my favorite places both on-line and in malls to order unusual kitchenware and gadgets. Their nonstick cast-iron sunflower cake pan is an excellent addition to my kitchen. **www.Williams-Sonoma.com,** 1-877-812-6235

Bob's Red Mill is a wonderful source for stone ground organic whole grains and flours. I have been grinding my own whole blanched almonds into a meal in my food processor for some time. However, I recently discovered their almond flour product and found that its use improved both the texture and flavor of my Lemon Almond Sponge Cake and Almond Anise Biscotti. **www.BobsRedMill.com,** 1-800-349-2173

index

abdominoplasty, 52–53, 56–59, 68
achiote-roasted turkey breast with
    chimichurri sauce, 184–86
almond:
  -anise biscotti, 220–22
  and chicken spread, curried, 113–14
  -crusted cheesecakes, individual, with
    black cherry compote, 242–43
  -lemon sponge cake, 197–99
ancho-guajillo (sauce):
  chicken simmered in *pollo acapulco*,
    165–66
  shrimp, 166
anise-almond biscotti, 220–22
apple crisp protein shake, 100
artichoke tartar sauce, salmon burgers with,
  141
asparagus, roasted, 240
avocado crema, spicy, Baja roasted chicken
  with, 167–68

Baja roasted chicken with spicy avocado
  crema, 167–68
banana bread:
  light, 219–20
  protein shake, 99
banana(s):
  chocolate-covered, protein shake, 99
  creamy, protein shake, 98
  frozen in protein shakes, 96
  nog, 98
  -orange frosted protein shake, 99
  Vermont, protein shake, 98
bariatric surgery:
  centers for, viii, ix–x, 13–14
  pre-op testing for, 62–63
  questions and answers about, 61–84
  types of, vii–viii, 61–62
beans, black, *see* black beans

beef tenderloin, garlic-herb, with roasted
  garlic cream, 239–40
Belgian chocolate cheesecake, 192–94
Bengal shrimp korma, 128–29
berry:
  coulis, orange panna cotta with,
    215–16
  see also specific berries
biscotti, almond-anise, 220–22
black beans:
  and red pepper sauté, jerk chicken with,
    161–62
  soup, creamy, 106–7
Bloody Mary's, ultimate, 236–37
blueberry(ies):
  cheesecake, 194–95
  fresh, with vanilla crème anglaise,
    213–14
Body Mass Index (BMI), 6–7
  in morbid obesity, 7, 8
bruschetta, salmon, 138–39
burgers:
  salmon, with artichoke tartar sauce,
    141–42
  turkey, with muffuletta salad, 186–87
burping, 81

café México protein shake, 100
cake(s):
  lemon-almond sponge, 197–99
  tangerine custard, 199–200
  see also cheesecakes; pies
calcium supplements, 76–78
Cancun sunset protein shake, 101
cannoli pudding, 212
carbohydrates, xiii, 40, 87–91
Carrasquilla, Carlos, vii–x, 9–10, 17, 23, 36
catfish with spicy orange sauce, 145–46
ceviche, shrimp, 134–35

cheese:
    log, teriyaki, 234
    puff, green chile, with roasted tomato salsa,
        118–19
cheesecake(s):
    Belgian chocolate, 192–94
    blueberry, 194–95
    individual almond-crusted, with black
        cherry compote, 242–43
cherry:
    black, compote, individual almond-crusted
        cheesecakes with, 242–43
    chocolate protein shake, 100
    clafouti, fresh, 216–17
    pie protein shake, 101
chicken, 157–80
    and almond spread, curried, 113–14
    Baja roasted, with spicy avocado crema,
        167–68
    cacciatore, 172–73
    chipotle salad, roasted, 160–61
    cutlets with sun-dried tomato dijon sauce,
        158–59
    with dijon-orange sauce, 164–65
    garlic roasted, with black olive tapenade,
        170–71
    jerk, with black bean and pepper sauté,
        161–62
    Marsala, 163–64
    paprikash, 176–78
    sauté Milanese, 171–72
    sesame roasted, 179–80
    simmered in ancho-guajillo sauce, *pollo
        acapulco*, 165–66
    stew with green chiles, *pollo chile verde*,
        174–75
    stock, 104–5
    tagine, 168–70
    tandoori, 178–79
    thighs, 157–58
    with tomato and feta sauce, 175–76
chiles, green, *see* green chiles
chipotle, roasted chicken salad, 160–61
chocolate:
    cheesecake, Belgian, 192–94
    cherry protein shake, 100
    -covered banana protein shake, 99
    cream crepes, 206–7
    genoise, 196–97
    Mexican, protein shake, 100
    pudding, Walker's favorite, 211
Christmas, menu for, 233–44
clafouti, fresh cherry, 216–17
clothing, exchanging of, 82–83
Coates, Penelope, 77

coconut:
    patty protein shake, 101
    toasted, custards, 204–5
coffee, panna cotta, 214–15
compote, black cherry, individual almond-
    crusted cheesecakes with, 242–43
cookies and cream protein shake, 98
cranberry sauce, 230
cream of potato soup, 105–6
cream puffs, 208–9
creamy banana protein shake, 98
creamy black bean soup, 106–7
crème anglaise, vanilla fresh blueberries with,
    213–14
crepes:
    chocolate cream, 206–7
    suzette, 205–6
crisp green onion and parmesan polenta
    cakes, 241–42
curried chicken and almond spread,
    113–14
custard(s):
    cakes, tangerine, 199–200
    spiced pumpkin, 217–18
    toasted coconut, 204–5
    vanilla egg, 117–18

desserts, 191–223
dijon:
    -orange sauce, chicken with, 164–65
    sun-dried tomato sauce, chicken cutlets
        with, 158–59
dip, pinto bean, 110–11
dumping syndrome, xiii, 5, 21, 40, 44, 45,
    59–60, 91–92

EAS Carb Control Shakes, 42, 54, 95
egg custard, vanilla, 117–18
eggnog, 244
Elvis's favorite protein shake, 98
exercise, after Gastric Bypass (RNY), 20, 22,
    33, 79

fennel and red pepper sauté, spiced tuna
    steaks with, 155–56
Fen-Phen, 3, 62
feta:
    Mykonos shrimp with, 127–28
    and tomato sauce, chicken with, 175–76
fish and seafood, 20, 22–23, 36, 125
    buying and preparing of, 125–26
    recipes for, 125–56
    see also specific fish
Florida Medical Center, surgical floor and
    bariatric suites at, 13–14, 17

flounder, simple, with salsa, 147–48
fool, strawberry, 210
French onion soup, 108–9
fresh blueberries with vanilla crème anglaise, 213–14
fresh cherry clafouti, 216–17
frittata, Sunday morning, 120–21
fruits:
  carbohydrates in, 90–91
  see also specific fruits

game hens:
  grandma's lemon, 181–82
  orange teriyaki, 180–81
garlic:
  -herb beef tenderloin with roasted garlic cream, 239–40
  roasted chicken with black olive tapenade, 170–71
  roasted vegetable sauté, creamy, turkey tenderloins with, 183–84
Gastric Bypass (RNY):
  author's journal before, 13–16
  author's journal following, 17–60
  candidates for, 4–5, 6–7, 8, 16
  celebrities opting for, 4–5, 8, 9
  choosing surgeon for, 8, 9–10
  cooking and eating after, 5–6, 10–11, 13, 14, 17, 18, 19, 20–21, 24, 30–31, 36, 38, 39–40, 52, 53, 55, 88, 102
  eating out after, 22–23, 25–28, 30–31, 34–35, 35–36, 37–38, 41, 42–45, 47, 48–50, 51–52, 59, 81–82
  family friction over, 32–33, 63
  food to eat in the weeks following, 66, 85, 88, 93–124
  as gold standard of bariatric surgery, vii, 7, 61
  health problems corrected by, viii, 7, 54
  last meals before, 13, 14, 16, 64–65
  lifestyle and self-image changes after, viii, 6, 18, 19, 20, 21, 23, 28–29, 32–33, 34, 35–36, 39, 40, 43, 46, 47, 48, 50–51, 55–56, 73–74
  pain and swelling after, 8, 17–18, 20, 21–22, 67–68, 83, 88
  post-operative anxieties about, xiii, 70, 71–72
  risks and side effects of, 7, 54–55
  stomach and intestines in, 1, 5–6, 7, 17, 22, 40, 48, 55, 61, 70, 80, 81, 88, 93
  techniques used in, 4, 7–8, 17
  traveling after, 41–51, 35–36, 54, 55–56
genoise, chocolate, 196–97
ginger-tahini sauce, halibut with, 154–55

grande sugar-free hazelnut latte protein shake, 99
grandma's lemon game hens, 181–82
green beans, Southern style, 228–29
green chile(s):
  cheese puff with roasted tomato salsa, 118–19
  chicken stew with, *pollo chile verde*, 174–75
  crema, roasted tilapia with, 146–47
green onion and parmesan polenta cakes, crisp, 241–42
grilled salmon with wasabi sauce, 144–45
grilled shrimp with romesco sauce, 130–31
grits and shrimp, Southern, 135–37
grouper, 125
  with red pepper coulis, 150
  roasted, with tomatoes and herbed cream sauce, 148–49
gurgles, 81

hair loss, 72–73
halibut with ginger-tahini sauce, 154–55
hazelnut sugar-free latte protein shake, grande, 99
holiday party menu for, 233–44
hospitals:
  equipped for bariatric surgery, viii, ix–x, 13–14
  items to pack for stay in, 65–66
hummus, 109–10

ice, strawberry Italian, 222–23
individual almond-crusted cheesecakes with black cherry compote, 242–43
insulin:
  carbohydrates and, 87
  dumping syndrome and, 91
insurance:
  bariatric surgery and, 64
  plastic surgery and, 53, 69
Italian ice, strawberry, 222–23
Italian meatballs, 189–90

jerk chicken with black bean and pepper sauté, 161–62

Laparoscopic Adjustable Gastric Band (Lap-Band), 61, 62
laparoscopic surgery, 4, 7–8, 17
lemon:
  -almond sponge cake, 197–99
  meringue pie, 202–3
light banana bread, 219–20
light manicotti, 122–24

mahimahi with puttanesca sauce, 151–52
mango:
  in protein shakes, 96, 97
  salsa, roasted salmon with, 143–44
manicotti, light, 122–24
meatball(s):
  Italian, 189–90
  soup, Mexican, 121–22
meatloaf, turkey mushroom, 188–89
Mediterranean tuna spread, 112–13
meringue pie, lemon, 202–3
Mexican chocolate protein shake, 100
Mexican meatball soup, 121–22
Milanese chicken sauté, 171–72
mochaccino protein shake, 99
mushroom turkey meatloaf, 188–89
mustard dressing, seared scallop salad with,
  137–38
Mykonos shrimp with feta, 127–28

nutrient deficiencies, 74–78

obesity:
  co-morbidities and, vii, 63
  as epidemic, vii
  humiliations of, 1–2, 35, 39, 56
  morbid, vii, 6–7, 8
olive, tapenade, black, garlic roasted chicken
  with, 170–71
onion:
  green, and parmesan polenta cakes, crisp,
    241–42
  roasted red, shrimp with tomatillo salsa
    and, 131–32
  soup, French, 108–9
orange:
  -banana frosted protein shake, 99
  -dijon sauce, chicken with, 164–65
  panna cotta with berry coulis, 215–16
  sauce, spicy catfish with, 145–46
  tangerine custard cakes, 199–200
  teriyaki game hens, 180–81

panna cotta:
  coffee, 214–15
  orange, with berry coulis, 215–16
panniculectomy, 52–53, 56–59, 68
papaya, in protein shakes, 96, 97
parmesan and crisp green onion polenta
  cakes, 241–42
peanut butter cup protein shake, 100
pecan(s):
  pie, amazing, 232
  spiced roasted, 235
pepper, red, *see* red pepper

Pereira, Jennifer, xi
pie:
  amazing pecan, 232
  lemon meringue, 202–3
  pumpkin, 231
  raspberry mousse, 201–2
pills, swallowing of, 78
pina colada protein shake, 101
pineapple, in protein shakes, 96, 97, 101
pinto bean dip, 110–11
pita chips, 110
plastic surgery, 52–53, 56–59, 68–69
polenta cakes, parmesan, crisp green onion
  and, 241–42
pollo acapulco, chicken simmered in ancho-
  guajillo sauce, 165–66
pollo chile verde, chicken stew with green
  chiles, 174–75
potato soup, cream of, 105–6
protein pudding treat, 116–17
protein(s), xiii, 75–76, 85–87
  determining correct amounts of,
    85–86
  foods, 86–87
  in quick meals, 79
  weight loss and, 86
protein shake(s), 21, 38, 93–101
  basic formula for, *see* shake formula,
    basic
  pantry ingredients for, 96–97
pudding:
  cannoli, 212
  protein treat, 116–17
  Walker's favorite, chocolate, 211
pumpkin:
  custard, spiced, 217–18
  pie, 231
puttanesca sauce, mahimahi with,
  151–52

ragù, turkey tomato, 115–16
raspberry:
  mousse pie, 201–2
  sauce, 193–94
red pepper:
  and black bean sauté, jerk chicken with,
    161–62
  coulis, grouper with, 150
  and fennel sauté, spiced tuna steaks with,
    155–56
roasted:
  asparagus, 240
  chicken chipotle salad, 160–61
  grouper with tomatoes and herbed cream
    sauce, 148–49

mahimahi with puttanesca sauce, 151–52
mango:
    in protein shakes, 96, 97
    salsa, roasted salmon with, 143–44
manicotti, light, 122–24
meatball(s):
    Italian, 189–90
    soup, Mexican, 121–22
meatloaf, turkey mushroom, 188–89
Mediterranean tuna spread, 112–13
meringue pie, lemon, 202–3
Mexican chocolate protein shake, 100
Mexican meatball soup, 121–22
Milanese chicken sauté, 171–72
mochaccino protein shake, 99
mushroom turkey meatloaf, 188–89
mustard dressing, seared scallop salad with,
    137–38
Mykonos shrimp with feta, 127–28

nutrient deficiencies, 74–78

obesity:
    co-morbidities and, vii, 63
    as epidemic, vii
    humiliations of, 1–2, 35, 39, 56
    morbid, vii, 6–7, 8
olive, tapenade, black, garlic roasted chicken
    with, 170–71
onion:
    green, and parmesan polenta cakes, crisp,
        241–42
    roasted red, shrimp with tomatillo salsa
        and, 131–32
    soup, French, 108–9
orange:
    -banana frosted protein shake, 99
    -dijon sauce, chicken with, 164–65
    panna cotta with berry coulis, 215–16
    sauce, spicy catfish with, 145–46
    tangerine custard cakes, 199–200
    teriyaki game hens, 180–81

panna cotta:
    coffee, 214–15
    orange, with berry coulis, 215–16
panniculectomy, 52–53, 56–59, 68
papaya, in protein shakes, 96, 97
parmesan and crisp green onion polenta
    cakes, 241–42
peanut butter cup protein shake, 100
pecan(s):
    pie, amazing, 232
    spiced roasted, 235
pepper, red, see red pepper

Pereira, Jennifer, xi
pie:
    amazing pecan, 232
    lemon meringue, 202–3
    pumpkin, 231
    raspberry mousse, 201–2
pills, swallowing of, 78
pina colada protein shake, 101
pineapple, in protein shakes, 96, 97, 101
pinto bean dip, 110–11
pita chips, 110
plastic surgery, 52–53, 56–59, 68–69
polenta cakes, parmesan, crisp green onion
    and, 241–42
pollo acapulco, chicken simmered in ancho-
    guajillo sauce, 165–66
pollo chile verde, chicken stew with green
    chiles, 174–75
potato soup, cream of, 105–6
protein pudding treat, 116–17
protein(s), xiii, 75–76, 85–87
    determining correct amounts of,
        85–86
    foods, 86–87
    in quick meals, 79
    weight loss and, 86
protein shake(s), 21, 38, 93–101
    basic formula for, see shake formula,
        basic
    pantry ingredients for, 96–97
pudding:
    cannoli, 212
    protein treat, 116–17
    Walker's favorite, chocolate, 211
pumpkin:
    custard, spiced, 217–18
    pie, 231
puttanesca sauce, mahimahi with,
    151–52

ragù, turkey tomato, 115–16
raspberry:
    mousse pie, 201–2
    sauce, 193–94
red pepper:
    and black bean sauté, jerk chicken with,
        161–62
    coulis, grouper with, 150
    and fennel sauté, spiced tuna steaks with,
        155–56
roasted:
    asparagus, 240
    chicken chipotle salad, 160–61
    grouper with tomatoes and herbed cream
        sauce, 148–49

flounder, simple, with salsa, 147–48
fool, strawberry, 210
French onion soup, 108–9
fresh blueberries with vanilla crème anglaise, 213–14
fresh cherry clafouti, 216–17
frittata, Sunday morning, 120–21
fruits:
    carbohydrates in, 90–91
    see also specific fruits

game hens:
    grandma's lemon, 181–82
    orange teriyaki, 180–81
garlic:
    -herb beef tenderloin with roasted garlic cream, 239–40
    roasted chicken with black olive tapenade, 170–71
    roasted vegetable sauté, creamy, turkey tenderloins with, 183–84
Gastric Bypass (RNY):
    author's journal before, 13–16
    author's journal following, 17–60
    candidates for, 4–5, 6–7, 8, 16
    celebrities opting for, 4–5, 8, 9
    choosing surgeon for, 8, 9–10
    cooking and eating after, 5–6, 10–11, 13, 14, 17, 18, 19, 20–21, 24, 30–31, 36, 38, 39–40, 52, 53, 55, 88, 102
    eating out after, 22–23, 25–28, 30–31, 34–35, 35–36, 37–38, 41, 42–45, 47, 48–50, 51–52, 59, 81–82
    family friction over, 32–33, 63
    food to eat in the weeks following, 66, 85, 88, 93–124
    as gold standard of bariatric surgery, vii, 7, 61
    health problems corrected by, viii, 7, 54
    last meals before, 13, 14, 16, 64–65
    lifestyle and self-image changes after, viii, 6, 18, 19, 20, 21, 23, 28–29, 32–33, 34, 35–36, 39, 40, 43, 46, 47, 48, 50–51, 55–56, 73–74
    pain and swelling after, 8, 17–18, 20, 21–22, 67–68, 83, 88
    post-operative anxieties about, xiii, 70, 71–72
    risks and side effects of, 7, 54–55
    stomach and intestines in, 1, 5–6, 7, 17, 22, 40, 48, 55, 61, 70, 80, 81, 88, 93
    techniques used in, 4, 7–8, 17
    traveling after, 41–51, 35–36, 54, 55–56
genoise, chocolate, 196–97
ginger-tahini sauce, halibut with, 154–55

grande sugar-free hazelnut latte protein shake, 99
grandma's lemon game hens, 181–82
green beans, Southern style, 228–29
green chile(s):
    cheese puff with roasted tomato salsa, 118–19
    chicken stew with, *pollo chile verde*, 174–75
    crema, roasted tilapia with, 146–47
green onion and parmesan polenta cakes, crisp, 241–42
grilled salmon with wasabi sauce, 144–45
grilled shrimp with romesco sauce, 130–31
grits and shrimp, Southern, 135–37
grouper, 125
    with red pepper coulis, 150
    roasted, with tomatoes and herbed cream sauce, 148–49
gurgles, 81

hair loss, 72–73
halibut with ginger-tahini sauce, 154–55
hazelnut sugar-free latte protein shake, grande, 99
holiday party menu for, 233–44
hospitals:
    equipped for bariatric surgery, viii, ix–x, 13–14
    items to pack for stay in, 65–66
hummus, 109–10

ice, strawberry Italian, 222–23
individual almond-crusted cheesecakes with black cherry compote, 242–43
insulin:
    carbohydrates and, 87
    dumping syndrome and, 91
insurance:
    bariatric surgery and, 64
    plastic surgery and, 53, 69
Italian ice, strawberry, 222–23
Italian meatballs, 189–90

jerk chicken with black bean and pepper sauté, 161–62

Laparoscopic Adjustable Gastric Band (Lap-Band), 61, 62
laparoscopic surgery, 4, 7–8, 17
lemon:
    -almond sponge cake, 197–99
    meringue pie, 202–3
light banana bread, 219–20
light manicotti, 122–24

salmon with mango salsa, 143–44
salmon with tzatziki sauce, 140–41
sweet potatoes, 229–30
tilapia with green chile crema, 146–47
turkey, 225–28
romesco sauce, grilled shrimp with, 130–31
Roux-en-Y Gastric Bypass procedure, *see*
    Gastric Bypass (RNY)

Sachse, Rainer, 52–53
salad:
    adding of, back to diet, 80, 103
    muffuletta, turkey burgers with, 186–87
    roasted chicken chipotle, 160–61
    salmon, 114–15
    seared scallop with mustard dressing,
      137–38
    shrimp spread, 111–12
salmon:
    baked in salsa verde, 139–40
    bruschetta, 138–39
    burgers with artichoke tartar sauce,
      141–42
    grilled, with wasabi sauce, 144–45
    roasted, with mango salsa, 143–44
    roasted, with tzatziki sauce, 140–41
    salad, 114–15
salsa:
    mango, roasted salmon with, 143–44
    roasted tomato, green chile cheese puff
      with, 118–19
    simple flounder with, 147–48
    tomatillo shrimp with roasted red onion
      and, 131–32
    verde, salmon baked in, 139–40
scallop salad with mustard dressing, seared,
    137–38
seafood, *see* fish and seafood; *specific fish*
sesame roasted chicken, 179–80
shake formula, basic, 97
    incredible shake variations to add to,
      98–101
shrimp:
    ancho-guajillo, 166
    ceviche, 134–35
    creole, 132–33
    with feta, Mykonos, 127–28
    grilled, with romesco sauce, 130–31
    and grits, Southern, 135–37
    korma, Bengal, 128–29
    Louis cocktail, 237–38
    with roasted red onion and tomatillo salsa,
      131–32
    salad spread, 111–12
simple flounder with salsa, 147–48

soda, drinking of, 80–81
soft foods, 18, 19, 24, 102–24
soup:
    chicken stock, 104–5
    cream of potato, 105–6
    creamy black bean, 106–7
    French onion, 108–9
    Mexican meatball, 121–22
    stracciatella, 103–4
Southern shrimp and grits, 135–37
Southern style green beans, 228–29
spiced:
    pumpkin custard, 217–18
    roasted pecans, 235
    roast turkey breast, 168
    tuna steaks with fennel and red pepper
      sauté, 155–56
sponge cake, lemon-almond, 197–99
staples, removed after Gastric Bypass, 17,
    18, 69
stock, chicken, 104–5
stracciatella, 103–4
strawberry:
    fool, 210
    Italian ice, 222–23
sugar, xiv, 11, 25–26, 28, 39
    dumping syndrome and, xiii, 21, 40, 44,
      45, 59–60, 91–92
Sunday morning frittata, 120–21
supplements, vitamin and mineral, 74–78
support groups, viii, ix, 39–40, 71–72, 73,
    82
sushi, 22–23, 125, 126
sweet potatoes, roasted, 229–30
swordfish:
    with charred tomato vinaigrette,
      152–53
    steaks with cilantro cream, 153–54

tagine, chicken, 16–70
tahini-ginger sauce, halibut with,
    154–55
tandoori chicken, 178–79
tangerine custard cakes, 199–200
tapenade, black olive, garlic roasted chicken
    with 170–71
teriyaki cheese log, 234
Thanksgiving, menu for, 225–232
thyroid problems, 33–34
tilapia, roasted, with green chile cream,
    146–47
toasted coconut custards, 204–5
tomato(es):
    dijon sun-dried, sauce, chicken cutlets
      with, 158–59

tomato(es) (*continued*)
    and feta sauce, chicken with, 175–76
    roasted grouper with herbed cream sauce
        and, 148–49
    salsa, roasted green chile cheese puff with,
        118–19
    turkey ragù, 115–16
    vinaigrette, charred, swordfish with,
        152–53
tropical dream protein shake, 101
tuna:
    spread, Mediterranean, 112–13
    steaks, spiced, with fennel and red pepper
        sauté, 155–56
turkey, 183–90
    breast, achiote-roasted, with chimichurri
        sauce, 184–86
    breast, spiced roast, 168
    burgers with muffuletta salad, 186–87
    mushroom meatloaf, 188–89
    roasted, 225–28
    tenderloins, with creamy roasted garlic
        vegetable sauté, 183–84
    tomato ragù, 115–16

ultimate Bloody Marys, 236–37

vanilla egg custard, 117–18
vegetable(s):
    carbohydrates in, 88–90
    first added back to meals, 80
    sauté, creamy roasted garlic, turkey
        tenderloins with, 183–84
    see also specific vegetables
Vermont banana protein shake, 98
Vertical Banded Gastroplasty (VBG), 61–62
vinaigrette, charred tomato, swordfish with,
    152–53
VistaVitamins, 75–76, 77–78
vomiting, 5, 7, 18, 23, 31, 36, 57, 81

Walker's favorite chocolate pudding, 211
water, drinking of, 54–55, 78–79
weight loss:
    diets and, 2–3
    gastric bypass and, viii, 7, 18, 20, 22, 23,
        24, 26, 27, 31, 32, 33, 35, 36, 37, 39, 40,
        43, 53, 61, 71, 72, 82–84
    protein and, 86
Wilson, Carnie, 4–5, 8, 9
Windham Bonaventure Spa, 28–30

Zero Carb Isopure, 21, 38, 93, 94